the**facts**

Multiple
Sclerosis

SANDRA AMOR

Professor, Pathology Department, VUMC,
Amsterdam, The Netherlands,
and
Queen Mary University of London,
London, UK

HANS VAN NOORT

Chief Scientific Officer, Delta Crystallon BV,
The Netherlands

OXFORD
UNIVERSITY PRESS

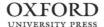
UNIVERSITY PRESS

Great Clarendon Street, Oxford OX2 6DP,
United Kingdom

Oxford University Press is a department of the University of Oxford.
It furthers the University's objective of excellence in research, scholarship,
and education by publishing worldwide. Oxford is a registered trade mark of
Oxford University Press in the UK and in certain other countries

British Library Cataloguing in Publication Data
Data available

Library of Congress Cataloging in Publication Data
Data available

ISBN 978-0-19-965257-0

Printed in Great Britain
on acid-free paper by
Ashford Colour Press Ltd, Gosport, Hampshire

the**facts**

Multiple
Sclerosis

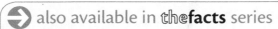
also available in **thefacts** series

ADHD, SECOND EDITION
Selikowitz
978-0-19-956503-0 | July 2009

Alzheimer's and other Dementias
Hughes
978-0-19-959655-3| August 2011

Angina and Heart Attack
Jevon
978-0-19-959928-8| November 2011

Asthma
Arshad
978-0-19-921126-5| October 2008

Autism and Asperger Syndrome
Baron-Cohen
978-0-19-850490-0 | May 2008

Breast Cancer
Saunders
978-0-19-955869-8 | June 2009

Depression, SECOND EDITION
Wasserman
978-0-19-960293-3 | October 2011

Down Syndrome, THIRD EDITION
Selikowitz
978-0-19-923277-2 | May 2008

Dyslexia and Other Learning
Difficulties, THIRD EDITION
Selikowitz
978-0-19-969177-7 | July 2012

Epilepsy, THIRD EDITION
Appleton
978-0-19-923368-7 | January 2009

Heart Disease
Chenzbraun
978-0-19-958281-5 | August 2010

Multiple Sclerosis
Amor
978-0-19-965257-0 | August 2012

Myotonic Dystrophy, SECOND EDITION
Harper
978-0-19-957197-0 | June 2009

Obsessive-Compulsive Disorder,
FOURTH EDITION
Rachman
978-0-19-956177-3 | March 2009

Osteoporosis
Black
978-0-19-921589-8 | February 2009

Panic Disorder, THIRD EDITION
Rachman
978-0-19-957469-8 | October 2009

Polycystic Ovary Syndrome
Elsheikh
978-0-19-921368-9 | January 2008

Post-traumatic Stress
Regel
978-0-19-956658-7 | April 2010

Pre-Natal Tests and Ultrasound
Burton
978-0-19-959930-1 | September 2011

Prostate Cancer, SECOND EDITION
Mason
978-0-19-957393-6 | June 2010

Pulmonary Arterial Hypertension
Handler
978-0-19-958292-1 | June 2010

Schizophrenia, THIRD EDITION
Tsuang
978-0-19-960091-5 | August 2011

Sexually Transmitted Infections,
THIRD EDITION
Barlow
978-0-19-959565-5 | March 2011

Sleep Problems in Children
and Adolescents
Stores
978-0-19-929614-9 | November 2008

The Pill and Other Forms of
Hormonal Contraception,
SEVENTH EDITION
Guillebaud
978-0-19-956576-4 | July 2009

Tourettes Syndrome, SECOND EDITION
Robertson
978-0-19-929819-8| October 2008

Preface

This book is about the biology of multiple sclerosis (MS), and is meant for people with MS, their families, carers, and other persons with an interest in MS. It is also intended for medical students, students in MS research, or established MS researchers who often focus on part of the story, but may find it useful to broaden their view.

Several useful books on MS are already available. Yet, most focus on the clinical or social side, or self-help strategies. While certainly of great help, such books often fall short in providing in-depth answers to more fundamental and general questions about the biology of MS. Information on this subject from more professional sources is often littered with strange terms, difficult to understand without specialist training. Information on the Internet tends to be fragmented and sketchy. In most cases, it is from untraceable or potentially biased sources, making it difficult to put everything together in a reliable way. In this book, we make an attempt to explain MS the way we understand it, as MS researchers.

Our inspiration comes from our experience with an award-winning initiative called 'Meet the Scientist', a forum to explain MS to people affected by the disease. It involves a booth at the UK MS Society's meetings where people can ask MS researchers anything about MS. This experience has taught us that many people with MS, and those around them, find it intriguing to hear more about the biology of MS. Getting to know more about the condition helps people to understand what to expect from having MS, and how they can manage it. Also, it may help them to judge whether newly advertised interventions or cures for MS have any merit.

This book addresses the most frequently asked questions on MS, and aims to provide some answers. We hope to have phrased the current ideas and information in a way that is accessible and balanced. We have done our best to avoid strange terms as much as possible. When we use them, we explain them. Of course, research continues, and some of the information in this book will go out of date. We certainly hope so. In due course, therefore, we aim to update this book, for it to remain a reliable source of up-to-date information.

We are indebted to our colleagues in MS research with whom we had so many discussions on the subject. We particularly thank Dr Monica Calado Marta and Professor Gavin Giovannoni for helping us summarize relevant medical and social information about MS in the second chapter of this book. We are also grateful to Elleke Meijer, Wouter van Noort, Sarah Webb, Robert Schoonenberg, Regina Peferoen-Baert, and Richard Verbeek, who have reviewed drafts of this book, and helped us improve it. If you as a reader should feel that additional areas need to be included or amended, please do not hesitate to let us know, since this book is ultimately for you.

Sandra Amor and Hans van Noort
June 2012

Contents

Contributors

Gavin Giovannoni
Professor of Neurology,
Neurosciences & Trauma Centre,
Queen Mary University of London,
Neurosciences, Blizard Institute,
London, UK

Monica Calado Marta
Clinical Research Fellow,
Neurosciences & Trauma Centre,
Queen Mary University of London,
Neurosciences, Blizard Institute,
London, UK

Glossary

Adaptive immune system: the collection of immune cells that respond very specifically, but initially slowly, to viruses and bacteria. After a first wave of response, some adaptive immune cells persist, making us immune to a particular microbe.

Antibodies: substances secreted by certain immune cells. They stick tightly to structures such as micro-organisms, but may also stick to parts of our own body. Antibodies mark their target for destruction by the immune system.

Antigen: a fragment of a micro-organism, tumour cell, or something from our own body, that is put on display by innate immune cells for recognition by adaptive immune cells.

Autoimmunity: immune reactions against something that belongs to our own body.

CCSVI: chronic cerebrospinal venous insufficiency. Restricted flow of blood away from the brain caused by partially blocked veins in the neck.

Central nervous system: brain, spinal cord, and the eye nerves.

Chromosome: a string of DNA containing many genes. We have two sets of 23 different chromosomes in our cells.

DNA: deoxyribonucleic acid. DNA is made of long strings of four different chemicals. The order of these chemicals encodes our genes, the building instructions of proteins.

EDSS: Expanded Disability Status Scale. A scale used by neurologists to express the severity of MS symptoms.

Epigenetic regulation: changes in the way genes are actually used by the body.

Gene: a segment of the DNA string, which contains the building instructions for a single protein.

Innate immune system: the collection of immune cells that respond quickly to invading micro-organisms or tumours, and help start adaptive immune reactions against these.

Macrophage: an innate immune cell that can be found almost everywhere in our body. It can quickly remove dangerous substances.

MHC protein: the substance used by innate immune cells to display fragments of viruses and bacteria to adaptive immune cells.

Microglia: the brain's macrophages.

MRI: magnetic resonance imaging. A technique to make scans of the brain during life, revealing where and when inflammation occurs.

MS lesion: the area in the brain or spinal cord where immune reactions damage the tissue during MS.

Myelin: the protective layer that surrounds nerve fibres.

Oligodendrocytes: cells in the brain and spinal cord that produce myelin.

Proteins: substances that are very active players in the body. They do most things, from building cells, producing fats and sugars, changing or breaking down other substances, to influencing chemical processes.

Relapse: an episode during which MS symptoms become more severe.

Remission: an episode during which MS symptoms become less severe.

Tolerance: immune cells not being bothered by what they bump into.

1

What is multiple sclerosis?

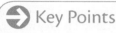

> ### Key Points
>
> ◆ Multiple sclerosis (MS) is caused by recurrent immune reactions in the brain and spinal cord. These reactions damage the tissue in such a way that nerve signals which run through those areas are weakened, or lost completely.
>
> ◆ Close examination of the brain shows that apart from localized immune reactions, other abnormalities are also seen in the central nervous system. It is quite likely that these actually provoke the immune reactions.

Multiple sclerosis, or MS, is a disease of the central nervous system. It involves the brain, spinal cord, and nerves of the eye. Nerves in the peripheral nervous system are not involved. In the central nervous system, the problem which keeps coming up in MS is the development of immune reactions. Similar to what happens in other immune reactions, large numbers of white blood cells go into the tissue and start to cause swellings, and even some damage to the tissue. The destruction of tissue in MS occurs only around nerve fibres. Why this is so, or why the immune reactions start in the first place, is currently not known. In the Western world, about 1 in 1000 people develops MS. Their numbers are increasing.

The tissue in brain and spinal cord may recover from the damage that the immune reactions cause but, unfortunately, it does not always. The signals that nerve fibres are supposed to pass on may therefore be temporarily hampered, but they may also be lost forever. Since those signals are crucial for controlling different functions in the body, each of those functions may be affected, dependent on where the damage occurs. In each person with MS, immune reactions may take place in different parts of the central nervous system, and with a different frequency or intensity. This makes MS difficult to recognize, and its course difficult to predict. There is no single set of symptoms that all people with MS have, nor is there any single way the disease develops over time. Most people with MS start to become troubled by it between the ages of 25 and 35. MS never goes away once it has started, but while in some people it may gradually cause serious problems, it can also remain quite mild in others.

What does MS look like?

To understand which symptoms can result from MS, it is useful to first see what the immune reactions in brain and spinal cord look like. While MS is about the brain, spinal cord, and nerves of the eye, we will focus on the brain here.

In the brain, the tissue can be roughly divided into two areas. The centre part is called the white matter, while the outside layer is called the grey matter, as illustrated in Fig. 1.1. The most important difference is that in the white matter all the nerve fibres are packed together, while in the grey matter the nerve cells themselves are located. Through their long fibres, they communicate with each other, and with the rest of the body (see Fig. 1.2). The area in the brain where the fibres run is white, because there is a white substance, called myelin, which covers and protects the nerve fibres (see Fig. 1.3). It is the same in the spinal cord, apart from the fact that the white matter is on the outside there.

In MS, the immune reactions develop exactly where myelin is found. This explains why the function of nerve cells is affected in MS—the protective

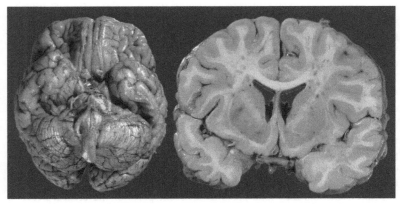

Fig. 1.1 A normal human brain, as seen from underneath (left). Inside the brain, the areas of white and grey matter can be seen (right).

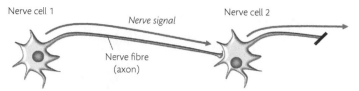

Fig. 1.2 Nerve cells communicate with each other through long fibres called axons, along which the nerve signal travels. Many signals eventually control the movement of muscles.

myelin layer is damaged by the immune reaction, and so is the nerve fibre that it surrounds. Although the myelin that protects nerve fibres is particularly abundant in white matter, it is also found in smaller amounts in grey matter, and immune reactions may also develop there. When looking at the brain of someone who had MS, the most striking feature is the presence of multiple greyish scars, mainly in the white matter (see Fig. 1.4). This feature has given MS its name. Multiple sclerosis means 'many scars'. These scars are the remains of tissue damaged by immune reactions. Just like scars in other parts of our body, they remain for life.

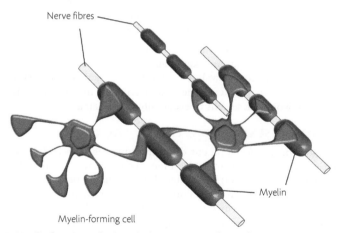

Fig. 1.3 Myelin-forming cells deposit their protective layer of myelin around the nerve fibres in the brain and spinal cord.

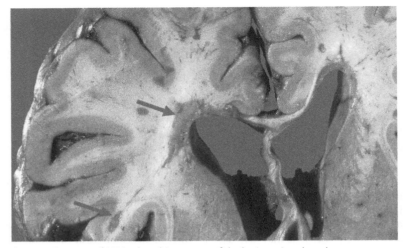

Fig. 1.4 The scars of MS in the white matter of the brain, pointed out by arrows.

MS under the microscope

By looking at brain tissue under a microscope, much more of the disease process can be revealed. We obviously cannot see under a microscope how a single spot changes as the immune reaction develops. Tissue samples can only provide snapshots of a single point in time. Yet, by looking at many different examples, it is possible to reconstruct the process.

It was long believed that the immune system attacks brain tissue in MS as a first step in the process. Careful examination of brains under the microscope, however, has changed this view. It is now becoming increasingly clear that the brain itself creates the problem. The brain itself calls in cells of the immune system, and provokes these cells to eventually cause damage.

The damage starts from within the brain

The first step in the development of an immune reaction in MS is not an immune attack by aggressive white blood cells. Instead, and well before immune cells from the blood have entered the brain, the brain cells that form myelin start to change. This causes other cells in the brain to respond to this change. The cells that form myelin are called 'oligodendrocytes', and the neighbouring cells that respond to their signals are called 'microglia'. Other types of brain cells with an important supportive function are called 'astrocytes', star-like cells. These cells also change their behaviour during MS.

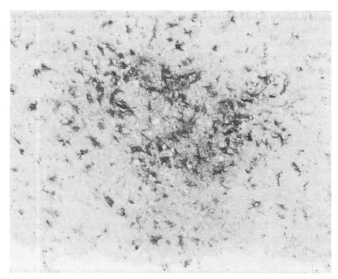

Fig. 1.5 The first step in the immune reaction that causes MS. Cells in the brain called 'microglia' to become activated, probably by signals from myelin-forming cells. Here, a microscopic image shows a thin slice of brain tissue, which is treated with chemicals that turns activated microglia dark. This reveals a cluster of such activated microglia in brain tissue. At this early stage, no immune cells from the blood are around yet.

Fig. 1.5 illustrates how, under a microscope, small areas can be seen in the brain of someone with MS in which microglia produce much more so-called MHC proteins than normal. Producing more of these MHC proteins is what microglia do when they become active. In the brain sample shown in Fig. 1.5, these proteins are stained dark with special chemicals, thus highlighting where activated microglial cells are. MHC proteins are very important as they allow an immune response to develop (more on this is explained in Chapter 5 on the immune system). Accumulation of MHC proteins on the surface of microglia is one of the first clearly visible steps in the process. What sets it off is probably a change in myelin-forming cells, which is subsequently recognized by neighbouring microglia. What exactly this change in myelin-forming cells is, or why it occurs, remains a mystery for the moment.

The immune system enters the stage

Next, the white blood cells that belong to the immune system enter the tissue. They are called in, not knowing what to expect. Instrumental in this step are the special blood vessel walls in the brain. Under normal conditions, blood vessel walls in brain and spinal cord are unusually tight. This is to prevent substances and cells in blood from entering our central nervous system too easily. We call the very tight blood vessel walls in brain and spinal cord the 'blood–brain barrier'. It is not like a brick wall, however. The vessel walls can pick up signals of danger or damage from within the brain itself. When they do, they respond by producing special proteins on the inside of the vessel wall, which can stick to immune cells that float by in the blood. A Velcro-like mechanism is used for this. The vessel wall proteins that appear in response to signs of danger or damage are somewhat like loops. Immune cells, on the other hand, carry proteins on their surface that may be compared to hooks. By using these hooks to attach to, vessel wall 'loop' proteins may catch immune cells floating by in blood, and guide them into the brain. The resulting accumulation of white blood cells around the vessel can be seen in Fig. 1.6. In this way, the brain and spinal cord can actively recruit immune cells from the bloodstream, when there is something unusual going on inside that may require an immune reaction. It appears that the brain and spinal cord affected by MS regularly give such recruitment signals.

When immune cells enter the brains of people with MS, some of those cells apparently come across a substance they feel should be attacked. Unfortunately, we still do not know for certain what that substance is. Since no one has ever

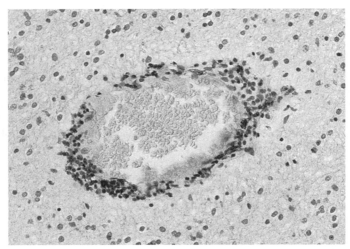

Fig. 1.6 Immune cells from the blood are called in by the brain and spinal cord in MS. Here, many such cells have worked their way in from a small blood vessel, in response to the call. The cores of these immune cells have been stained dark to make them visible under the microscope.

found a bacterium or virus to explain the immune reaction, we assume there must be a natural substance in the brain which causes it. This is why MS is referred to as an 'autoimmune disease'. It means that the immune system appears to turn against something in the body. This does not mean that the immune system causes MS, but it does mean that it is instrumental in creating the damage. It is like the fuel in cars—having a full tank does not immediately make a car speed away, but the fuel is nevertheless essential for driving once the engine has started. In fact, and as discussed later on in more detail, the immune system in people with MS—the fuel for the immune reaction—appears to be largely normal. Yet it is provoked by problems that occur in the brain and spinal cord itself. The way the immune system responds in people with MS is pretty much what would happen in any other person, but only in people with MS does the provocation occur. This is important to keep in mind. Stories about MS often start by suggesting that it is caused by an autoimmune attack on the central nervous system. This is somewhat misleading. It is very likely that it is the brain itself that sets off MS, not the immune system.

The damage starts

Next, and provoked by the brain, a rather powerful immune reaction develops and starts to damage the tissue. This is an MS lesion, as shown in Fig. 1.7. As the MS lesion 'eats' through the tissue, the protective myelin cover of nerve

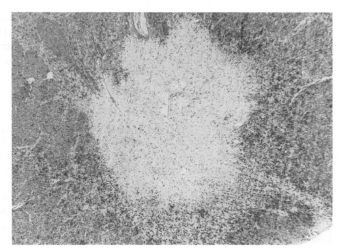

Fig. 1.7 The active immune reaction in the brain grows, and destroys myelin in its path. This is called an MS lesion. Myelin in the image is stained dark, thus showing how it is destroyed in the centre of the lesion. The cores of immune cells are also stained dark, revealing their presence in the destruction zone, at the edge of the lesion.

fibres gets stripped away and the nerve fibres themselves become damaged too. Finally, the reaction comes to an end. The MS lesion burns out and, similar to what happens, for example, in the skin, damaged tissue turns into a scar. Brain cells called astrocytes are largely responsible for this. Where nerve fibres once ran, astrocytes forming a scar have taken their place. Since a scar is just a filling substance, but does not pass on any nerve signals, this part of the brain or spinal cord is no longer functional.

This scenario applies to immune reactions in MS most of the time. However, as the process of lesion formation starts within the brain, it can still turn back to full recovery at the very early stages, but once white blood cells become activated and start to attack, the damage becomes largely irreversible. Still, signs of repair are observed even after myelin has been destroyed. This shows that the brain has made attempts to produce new layers of myelin around nerve fibres. These newly formed layers, however, tend to be thinner than the original ones, and appear to be more susceptible to any new immune reaction. In other situations where myelin is damaged by immune reactions, for example, after a viral infection in the brain, full repair seems to be the rule rather than the exception. Therefore the brain can indeed repair itself by making new layers of myelin when this becomes necessary, yet this repair system somehow does not work in MS. It is not fully clear why this is.

Careful studies using the microscope revealing this chain of events have also shown that the damage may look slightly different from one person to another. This is perhaps not unexpected, since people generally develop diseases in slightly different ways. Their genes differ, their immune systems differ, and their brains differ. It is not surprising, therefore, that variations exist in the immune reactions during MS. Yet, they all seem to follow the described basic pattern.

MRI scans

Using the microscope we can get some idea of what the immune reaction looks like. We can also use another method, called 'magnetic resonance imaging', commonly referred to as 'MRI'. The technology is somewhat complicated, but the basic idea is rather straightforward. MRI uses a very strong magnetic field to influence certain atoms in tissues. By having a charge and spinning around very fast, these atoms themselves act like tiny magnets. Like any other pair of magnets influences each other's position, the MRI machine does so with atoms in brain tissue. After making them spin, the MRI machine records how quickly the tiny atomic magnets in our brain return to their normal position. An immune reaction, swelling, or tissue damage changes the speed at which this happens. By recording this change for the various parts of the brain, and reflecting it in an image called the 'MRI scan', the machine shows where things are different from normal. Also, a leaky blood–brain barrier can be visualized, by using a contrast fluid called gadolinium. An intact blood–brain barrier blocks gadolinium from going into the brain, but a leaky one lets it pass. If gadolinium is injected into the bloodstream just before a scan is made, its appearance in the brain therefore indicates that blood vessels in that area have become leaky. This is another sign of the presence of an immune reaction. In different ways, an MRI scan can therefore tell us whether there is something going on, and exactly where. Examples of such scans are shown in Fig. 1.8.

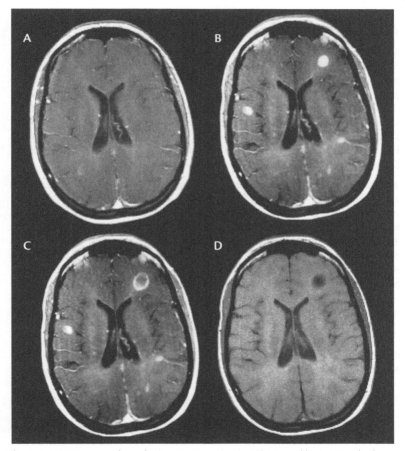

Fig. 1.8 MRI scans can show the immune reaction in MS. Normal brain tissue looks rather dark on such a scan (A), an immune reaction lights up (B), and progresses as a destructive ring (C). At the end of the process, a dark scar remains (D). The butterfly-like shape in the middle is formed by the brain ventricles, hollow spaces filled with brain fluid. The white rim reflects the skull.

While individual cells cannot be seen using an MRI scanner, the great advantage is that the process of inflammation and damage can be monitored in real time, making it possible to follow it in a person with MS as it actually happens. Repeated scans of people with MS have given us the same basic idea of the process as the microscopic pictures did. Also in MRI scans, some faint signals of change appear in brain tissues even before the blood vessels become leaky and damage develops. Again, this indicates that the brain itself starts the whole process.

How often do immune reactions develop?

MRI scans have revealed that immune reactions in the brains of people with MS develop surprisingly frequently. When scans are repeatedly made, over periods of months, for example, the MRI signals of MS lesions continuously come and go. This is particularly so in the early years of MS. As time passes, the signals appear less frequently. Episodes of real problems, the way people with MS themselves experience them, are called relapses. They tend to occur about once a year, or even less frequently. MRI signals revealing immune reactions in the brain appear about ten times more frequently than relapses. Clearly, not all the damage seen on MRI scans causes relapses.

The fact that MRI signals appear more frequently than clinical relapses poses a problem. It is obviously helpful to monitor MS with a scanner over time, for example, to see the effects of a new drug or intervention. The MRI scans can tell us relatively quickly and objectively whether any effect occurs. The scans are also helpful in predicting the future burden of disease symptoms in groups of people. Still, the real problem for people with MS is not the outcome of a scan, but the clinical symptoms they experience. There is a marked difference between the two. For this reason, MRI scans can still not be used on their own to keep track of how MS develops, without looking at what the person in question feels too. It would ignore what matters most.

Further reading

Compston A and Coles A (2008) Multiple sclerosis. *Lancet* **372**: 1502–17.

Franklin, RJM and ffrench-Constant C (2008) Remyelination in the CNS; from biology to therapy. *Nat Rev Neurosci* **9**: 839–55.

Van der Valk P and Amor S (2009) Preactive lesions in multiple sclerosis. *Curr Opin Neurol* **22**: 207–13.

2

What does it mean to have MS?

Monica Marta and Gavin Giovannoni

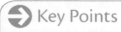 Key Points

- The impact of MS on people's lives is variable, and difficult to predict. Different functions of the body can become affected, and with varying severity. MS symptoms also often fluctuate over time.
- MS can also cause psychological problems, and affect relationships, social life, and work.
- There are several different ways to manage the individual symptoms or consequences of MS, apart from taking special MS drugs. A personalized approach with help from different types of healthcare professionals generally works best.

The symptoms of MS

In different people with MS, the damage caused by the inflammation may well occur in different parts of the brain and spinal cord. For this reason, one person with MS may experience problems that another person might never be troubled by. The severity of symptoms may also be very different from one person to another. Such symptoms may range from being almost unnoticeable to severe, and anything in between. In fact, quite a few people with MS do not show any clear signs of their condition at all to untrained eyes. Paradoxically, this in itself can be a cause of problems too. Family members and colleagues may sometimes think that complaints may be exaggerated, or even imaginary.

Society can sometimes be quite impatient with people who need special attention but still appear to be largely okay from the outside, especially when they are young.

Problems caused by MS often include blurred or double vision, weakness and stiffness, fatigue, numbness or tingling in limbs, problems in walking and maintaining balance. Over time, use of the legs may become increasingly difficult, necessitating the use of a cane, or eventually a wheelchair. It is good to stress that certainly not all people with MS will require wheelchair assistance. Two-thirds of people with MS remain quite able to walk for at least 15 years, and may only occasionally need supporting canes, crutches, or a wheelchair when their MS temporarily gets worse. Speech and swallowing can be impaired by MS as well. Other frequent symptoms include sexual problems, and loss of bladder control. Persistent pain and muscle stiffness, tremors, or spasticity may occur, as well as dizziness, vertigo, and tremor. Also so-called cognitive functions can be affected, things like memory and learning, or finding the right words to express oneself. People's mood can change, and they might start to feel anxious or depressed. Indeed, a wide range of issues can emerge, reflecting the wide variety of important things that the central nervous system controls. Later on in this chapter we will get back to some of these issues, and suggest ways to help manage them.

The general course of MS over time

The course of MS can also differ substantially between people, making it difficult to accurately predict for any given person what to expect. Especially during the first years of having MS, the symptoms of the condition often come and go. This coming and going of symptoms is called 'relapsing–remitting', and it is seen in about 85% of all people with MS. In this large group that experience relapses and remissions of symptoms, the majority will at some point get to the stage where remissions become less clear. At this stage, on average 10–20 years after diagnosis, the symptoms gradually become persistent. Relapses become less frequent, but recovery from these episodes of worsening no longer occurs. This stage of MS is referred to as 'secondary progressive'. In a much smaller group of about 15%, MS takes a course referred to as 'primary progressive'. It means that from the very start, disease symptoms gradually accumulate without clear relapses or episodes of improvement.

It is still not clear what makes MS develop in these different forms. No evidence has been found that there is something fundamentally different going on in people with the different patterns of symptoms. For example, when brain samples from people with different forms of MS are examined under a microscope, they all look pretty much the same. Still, certain therapies do not seem to work as well for primary-progressive MS as they may do for relapsing–remitting MS. The challenge remains to find out exactly why.

The diagnosis of MS

Clearly, the variable symptoms of MS do not make it easy for anyone to quickly recognize MS. Especially in the early stages, MS in one person can look quite different from MS in another person. Also the relatively low frequency of MS in the general population does not help people in the first line of healthcare, such as general practitioners, to become familiar with the condition. Most of them will encounter it only a few times in their career. There is also no simple test to establish whether someone has MS. There is nothing we can measure in blood or urine, for example, that can tell us so. This makes diagnosing MS difficult.

To make a diagnosis of MS, three things are important. The first is that the person must have signs of damage in at least two different places in the central nervous system. It is referred to as 'dissemination in space'. This can be established by an MRI scan, or by the fact that two different body functions are affected. A neurological problem that involves only one function, or the appearance of only one MS-like lesion on a MRI scan, could still be caused by something else. A single episode of a MS-like symptom is referred to as a 'clinically isolated syndrome'.

A second crucial factor in the diagnosis of MS is that the neurological problem or the MRI lesion is not an isolated event, but repeatedly occurs at least 1 month apart. The recurrent nature of MRI signals and clinical symptoms defines MS, so that must be also established. This is called 'dissemination in time'. Finally, other explanations for the symptoms must be ruled out. Other diseases such as, for example, some viral or bacterial infections, can sometimes cause symptoms similar to MS. Clearly, MRI scans are very helpful in making a diagnosis. After all, MRI signals come and go much more frequently than clinical relapses, as they also show inflammation that does not necessarily result in visible symptoms. Over the past years, the set of diagnostic criteria for MRI scans pointing to MS have been regularly refined, and the time it now takes to establish with reasonable certainty that someone has MS is much shorter than it used to be. Nowadays, even a single MRI scan can, in some cases, provide enough information to diagnose MS.

Apart from a general neurological examination and MRI scans, additional tests can be carried out to help diagnosis. This is especially important for diagnosing the primary progressive form of MS which lacks clear relapses. One of the more traditional tests relies on a spinal tap to obtain the fluid which bathes the brain and spinal cord. This fluid is examined for the presence of antibodies, called 'oligoclonal' antibodies. If present in the spinal tap, but not in blood, they are a strong indicator of MS (see Fig. 2.1 for an example). More than 95% of people with MS have these antibodies in spinal fluid. Although the antibodies may sometimes also emerge for other reasons, and

CSF   Serum   CSF   Serum

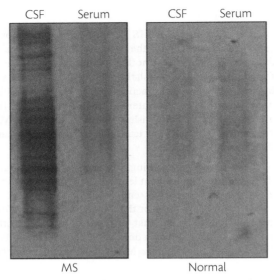

MS   Normal

Fig. 2.1 In almost everyone with MS, the fluid which surrounds the brain and spinal cord contains abnormal antibodies. This fluid, called cerebrospinal fluid, or CSF, is collected by a spinal tap. Here the antibodies are stained dark after having been separated in an electric field. They are not found in blood.

while it is still unclear what their significance actually is, they are a useful additional clue that we are dealing with MS.

Problems with the eyes and vision develop remarkably frequently in people with MS. About half the people with MS will at some point suffer from an inflamed eye nerve (known as the optic nerve, as shown in Fig. 2.2). In about one in five people, this is actually the first sign of their condition. An inflamed eye nerve can cause blurred vision, changes in colour perception, pain, and sometimes even blindness. Because of this frequent link between MS and problems with vision, additional diagnostic tests for MS focus on the eye. Diagnosis can be supported by a test of what is called 'visual evoked potential' or VEP. In this test, a person is asked to look at signals displayed on a TV-screen. When the eye sees the signal, it is rapidly passed on to the brain. The normal speed at which this happens is about 400 km/hour. In people with MS whose eye nerve is affected, the speed is reduced. By measuring how fast the signal travels, a neurologist can therefore gain additional confidence about a diagnosis of MS.

Another test focuses on thinning of the eye nerves, which is often seen in people with MS. Using a technique called 'optical coherence tomography', or OCT, thinning of the eye nerve can be measured. OCT is similar to the

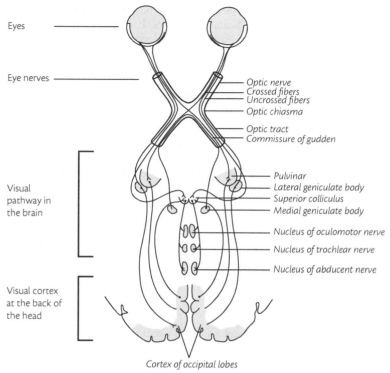

Eyes

Eye nerves

Optic nerve
Crossed fibers
Uncrossed fibers
Optic chiasma

Optic tract
Commissure of gudden

Pulvinar
Lateral geniculate body
Superior colliculus
Medial geniculate body

Nucleus of oculomotor nerve

Nucleus of trochlear nerve

Nucleus of abducent nerve

Visual
pathway in
the brain

Visual cortex
at the back of
the head

Cortex of occipital lobes

Fig. 2.2 Signals from the eyes need to travel all the way to the visual cortex at the back of the head, where they are finally translated into an image. MS often affects the nerves of the eye, and also brain regions through which the signals of the eye nerves travel As a result, people with MS often have problems with vision. (Reprinted from John Gray, *Anatomy of the Human Body* (1918), Figure 722, with permission of Elsevier.)

well-known ultrasound techniques used to obtain three-dimensional (3D) images of unborn babies. Instead of using the reflection of ultrasound waves, however, OCT uses reflections of light waves to create a 3D image of the eye and its nerve tracts. In this way, the thickness of eye nerves can be accurately measured. Diagnostic tools for MS such as OCT may help shorten the time required for diagnosis, so that treatment can be started as soon as possible.

Measuring MS

Having an objective way to express the severity of MS in numbers is very useful, for example, to see if a novel therapy tested during a trial is effective or not.

Two scales are often used to measure MS. The first is what is called the 'Expanded Disability Status Scale', or EDSS. It is illustrated in Fig. 2.3. The EDSS allows neurologists to measure the extent to which bodily functions are affected by MS. The second is the 'Multiple Sclerosis Impact Scale', or MSIS-29. This scale focuses on the patient's own perception of the impact that MS has on their daily activities, and on how they feel. Other scales are also used, but these two scales are widely accepted as a good way to measure MS, and they are often used in clinical trials.

The EDSS score is based on neurological testing of a wide range of different functional systems of the body. These include, for example, the ability to walk, coordination between different parts of the body such as between eyes and hands, touch and pain perception, speech and swallowing, bowel and bladder function, visual function, and mental state. On a scale from 0 to 10, the neurologist expresses the extent to which MS has affected these functions. When symptoms are relatively mild, and a variety of different functions may be affected, calculating an EDSS score is rather complicated. As disease progresses, higher EDSS scores become easier to determine as the EDSS system increasingly focuses on the ability to walk. Clearly, when a score is largely determined by someone's ability to walk 100 metres or take a few steps

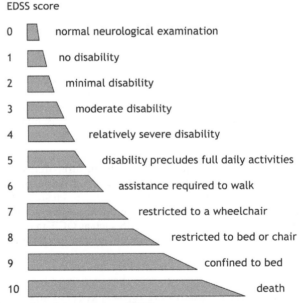

EDSS score

0	normal neurological examination
1	no disability
2	minimal disability
3	moderate disability
4	relatively severe disability
5	disability precludes full daily activities
6	assistance required to walk
7	restricted to a wheelchair
8	restricted to bed or chair
9	confined to bed
10	death

Fig. 2.3 Impression of the meaning of EDSS scores.

without any assistance, scoring is easy. There is, however, an obvious limit-ation to a scoring system which places such a strong emphasis only on walking, when it comes to evaluating something as complex as MS. There is much more to MS than just walking problems. Another limitation of the EDSS system is that it is not really linear. Having an EDSS score twice as high as some else's, does not mean that MS is twice as bad. It is not easy to compare the severity of walking or coordination problems with the severity of other symptoms such as sexual problems or fatigue, for example.

The second scoring system is based on the MSIS-29 scale, which is based on a questionnaire. By answering 29 questions, people with MS themselves rate the extent to which MS affects their life. Some questions cover the same body functions as addressed in the EDSS scoring system. They are about the func-tioning of arms and legs, balance and coordination, bladder control, fatigue, etc. Importantly, the questionnaire also addresses feelings and mental state, and the impact of MS on social and leisure activities. People with MS are also asked whether they feel their condition causes sleeping problems, lack of con-fidence, anxiety, or worries. The impact of MS on each of the 29 issues is given a score between 1 (no impact at all) and 5 (extreme impact). In this way, the MSIS-29 quantifies the extent to which people experience the impact of MS themselves. There are clearly aspects in which the MSIS-29 does more justice to the real impact of MS than the EDSS scoring system. For someone using a computer all day, problems with vision may have a very high impact. For someone else engaged in practical activities, problems with walking and maintaining balance may be more important. The MSIS-29 scoring system reflects these differences, and is therefore a very useful addition to the neurologist's objective EDSS system to measure MS.

Managing the symptoms of MS

Further on in this book, we will discuss several of the current options to slow down the activity and progression of MS with special MS drugs, or non-con-ventional approaches. Apart from those options, however, additional strategies exist to specifically address some of the separate symptoms that can be caused by MS. It is again important to stress that individual people with MS will not be confronted with all of the symptoms discussed here. They are issues encountered in large groups of people with MS, but they are not all problems that any single person with MS will necessarily get. For anyone just diagnosed with MS, is it therefore advisable to first talk with a well-informed person such as a specialized MS neurologist or MS nurse. They can help clarify each per-son's own form of MS, and demystify some of the problems generally asso-ciated with the condition. They can also help establish whether certain health issues are indeed caused by MS, or may actually be unrelated, and require separate intervention. After all, having MS does not mean that from then on all health issues are caused by it. Neurological issues probably are, but hypertension, diabetes, and infections, for example, may occur in someone with MS just as much as in anyone else, and require separate treatment.

Bladder dysfunction affects about 75% of people with MS. Problems may include urinary incontinence, feeling an urgent need to go to the toilet very frequently, excessive night urination, incomplete bladder emptying, or difficulties in passing urine. Avoiding dietary substances which stimulate urine formation, such as caffeine or alcohol, may help in such cases. Also pelvic floor exercises, or timed and regular voiding, can help alleviate some of the problems. While excessive urination can be reduced by some drugs, these do tend to increase the risk of urinary tract infections. For this reason, it is important to have the bladder inspected, for example, by ultrasound testing, before starting such medication. People who cannot completely empty their bladder may need the assistance of a small tube which can be passed along the bladder canal. Such a tube is called a catheter, and both women and men can be taught to use it themselves. People with advanced bladder problems may benefit from a permanent catheter. This requires an invasive procedure but it does avoid the high risk of a bladder infection which comes with handling a tube yourself. Another alternative is Botox®. It is a muscle relaxant which can be injected into the muscles that open the bladder. In this case, a tube is always required to help the relaxed muscles release urine.

Bowel dysfunction is also not uncommon in people with MS. Most times, it involves constipation. Dietary changes, such as increasing the intake of fluids and dietary fibres, may be very helpful in this case. Adhering to a steady rhythm of healthy meals and exercise also tends to help a lot. Laxatives should always be taken with care. Strategies to deal with the much rarer situation of bowel incontinence are best discussed with a doctor or MS nurse.

About half the people with MS experience *sexual problems*. Such problems may be in part caused by damage to the nerves that are involved in the controlling erection, ejaculation, and orgasm. In addition, other MS symptoms such as muscle weakness, fatigue, spasticity, and loss of sensation may easily interfere with a person's sex life. For women, difficulties in attaining an orgasm and a reduced libido are generally the main issues. For men, having and maintaining an erection is the main problem. Several drugs can help alleviate erectile problems in men, and in some cases arousal impairment in women. They include sildenafil (Viagra®), tadalafil (Cialis®) or alprostadil. Apart from physical issues, MS often also comes with psychological problems which may get in the way of enjoying intimacy and sex. Especially in the latter case, open and trustful communication between partners is important to find ways to manage sexual problems and to improve the situation.

Speech and swallowing impairment arise from damage to the nerves that control these functions. The melody of the speech typically becomes flatter, and people may start slurring. Clearly, these problems can greatly interfere with social interactions and work. In such cases, traditional speech therapy can be of benefit. Most people can be successfully trained to improve their speech rhythm and enunciation, and to limit slurring and the use of nasal sounds. Coughing or choking when eating and drinking, and unexplained chest infections, are frequent signs of swallowing problems. Again, a speech therapist may be helpful in such cases, to improve posture while eating and drinking, for example. Other helpful behavioural changes may include refraining from talking while eating, chewing only small portions, and consciously swallowing more than once per bite.

Cognitive impairment occurs in most people with MS. Slowing down of thinking, retrieving memories, or reasoning, and difficulties in concentration are clear signs of such impairment. It is not easy to fight against cognitive impairment, but a few things can still be done to help alleviate some of the problems caused by it, and to slow down its progression. Memory aids, or organizational aids, may help people avoid recurrent problems with daily activities and duties that are due to memory problems, for example. If anything helps to stop cognitive problems from getting worse, it is physical exercise. It is therefore advisable for people with MS to continue with physical activities as much as possible, and stay active. It does not always require heavy duty exercises. Simple stretching or balancing exercises for example are very useful too. The http://www.stayingsmart.org.uk website supported by the MS Trust gives useful explanations and examples of ways to deal with cognitive dysfunction.

Many people with MS experience feelings of *depression*, especially when pain or fatigue is in play as well. Since mental health is of key importance to our quality of life, addressing signs of depression is very important. Addressing depression in time is important to improve other MS symptoms, adherence to any form of therapy or treatment, and to reduce the risk of suicide. Depression associated with MS can be dealt with by antidepressive drugs, cognitive behaviour therapy, or a combination of both. Apart from such measures, personal strategies may often be of particular use. They may include a conscious approach to maintain and develop personal relationships with family and friends. Many find it useful to participate in support groups which help people with similar conditions to integrate, rather than be left on their own with their feelings. For others, keeping up with the latest news from science and medicine, or reading books such as this one, may help to empower themselves, meet new people, and to discover new opportunities. Like cognitive problems, depression can also be counteracted by regular physical and mental exercise.

Fatigue is a rather common symptom of MS, and in many cases, it is one of the more challenging ones. It is invisible, and for this reason, often difficult to appreciate for others. People with MS themselves describe it as having 'a bad flu', 'a curtain over the brain', or 'a small reservoir of energy that needs to be refilled much more often than before'. Fatigue is not the normal state of feeling tired, which disappears after a good night's rest. Fatigue does not disappear, and is still there the next morning. There are many possible causes. Fatigue can be a symptom of a new relapse developing, or may be caused by infections. Some people with MS becomes fatigued by heat, excess caffeine, certain drugs such as steroids, frequently going to the bathroom at night, pain, anxiety or depression, or being overweight. Chronic pain and spasms are frequently also associated with fatigue. Ways to combat fatigue are equally diverse, and include cognitive behavioural therapy, cardiovascular exercise, stretching and balance training, healthy meals, regular naps, and careful task planning. People with MS can often do themselves a favour by carefully selecting the best time of the day for important activities, and to space demanding activities over the week. Drug treatments for fatigue include amantadine, modafinil (which is also used to treat narcolepsy), and stimulating antidepressants such as fluoxetine.

As a result of the different symptoms as just described, especially when they are more severe, people with MS can also experience *secondary problems*. Managing these is obviously also important. We already mentioned urinary tract infections, which may become more frequent as the result of difficulties in releasing urine. Drop foot is another. When movement is impaired, people with MS may become overweight, develop pressure sores, or become troubled by osteoporosis more easily than others. Obesity, in turn, is a risk factor for diabetes. Also for these reasons, therefore, managing the symptoms as much as possible is important. This is particularly important for infections, as these drive the immune system to a stage of high alert, thus increasing the likelihood of relapses occurring.

Social aspects of MS

MS often has considerable consequences for family relationships, employment, and economic earning potential. Quite often, these consequences are more serious than would be expected on the basis of the actual impact of MS on people's physical abilities. Fear for what might happen may often be worse than what actually turns out to happen.

Since MS often affects young people, children, hereditary risks, and pregnancy are obvious issues of concern. Having children is an important part of many people's lives. As explained in more detail in another chapter, the risk of passing MS on to children is very small. It is probably reasonable to say that the hereditary risk is so small that it should not affect anyone's wish to have children. Being pregnant as such is also not an issue. In fact, MS symptoms tend to spontaneously improve, and fewer relapses occur during pregnancy. Changes in the hormonal balance during pregnancy are believed to cause these effects. In the period immediately after the baby is born, however, the relapse rate tends to increase again. In the long run, pregnancy appears to make no difference on the way MS develops. While common MS drugs have not yet shown any negative effects on babies, stopping such drugs during pregnancy is nevertheless always advised. Another factor to perhaps consider is the stability of relationships in which one of the partners has MS. This stability is considerably less than average. The rate of divorce is double that of the population, in particular when women are affected.

For most people, employment is not only a means to gain financial independence, but also an important source of social contacts, and a way to gain identity and a sense of value. After a diagnosis of MS, it is therefore important that people should aim to stay active and in full employment. It is advisable to inform the employer and others in the working place of possible changes, and explain what MS is really about. If necessary, adaptations may be discussed, such as improving the working environment, increasing flexibility in duties, or create possibilities to take some time off when needed. At the same time, however, it is useful to clarify to all those involved that while fatigue, cognitive impairment, and mobility may start to pose issues at some point, such symptoms need not necessarily stop someone from doing their work altogether. MS symptoms often prove to be temporary. After a relapse, and taking a step back for a while, resuming normal work could prove quite possible in many cases. Unemployment affects too many people with MS, at a level of about 50%. It is useful to keep in mind that unemployment and depression are linked. Unemployment aggravates depression, and it is more difficult for depressed people to go back to work. The best strategy to avoid this is to make the employer and colleagues fully aware of the situation, and keep on working as much as possible.

What to expect from the future?

Clearly, having been diagnosed with MS provokes many questions. While this chapter has hopefully answered quite a few of these, several might well remain. What most people with MS probably want to know more than anything is their personal prognosis. What to expect from the future? Unfortunately, it is almost impossible to provide anyone with MS with a reliable prediction of what to expect from their condition. This is actually one of the more difficult things to cope with. Not knowing what is going to happen next is a major part of having MS. Planning work, leisure activities, or holidays is no longer straightforward. Yet, having relapses more than a year apart, and experiencing full recovery from the symptoms after having had one, are generally good signs. In general, young women do better than others.

In this context, people might also wonder whether or not MS is a deadly condition. It almost never is. Only extremely rare and aggressive forms of MS can directly cause death. For the vast majority of people with MS, it is a chronic disease which may hamper them, but should not stop them from living on. Because of complications such as infections, poor mental health, metabolic or cardiovascular disease, and other consequences of long-standing disability, the average life expectancy is reduced by 10 years as compared to others.

After having stated this, we would immediately like to add a note. Options to manage and modify the course of MS have improved over recent years, and they will continue to improve. For this reason, data on how MS has impacted on people in the past have only limited predictive value. New MS drugs slow down progression more efficiently than old ones. More drugs will follow. For the futures of people with MS, this means that their prospects to keep MS under control will significantly improve. In addition, our understanding of MS continuously improves. We now know that relatively simple things that people with MS could do themselves, increases the likelihood that MS remains more under control than in the past. Eating healthy food, doing exercises, keeping a steady rhythm in daily activities, and fostering social contacts are all helpful. Further on in this book, we will discuss at least one additional and very simple lifestyle change which may really help. It is about the beneficial effects of vitamin D. Now knowing all this, and acting on it, might very well already make quite a difference.

For other questions about their personal condition, people with MS are best off with an MS specialist. In the UK, most people with MS will be put in contact with a MS nurse. They will be able to advise on who are suitable MS neurologists to consult. Reliable websites, such as the sites listed at the end of this book, will also tell you also about centres that run clinical trials. Such trials are run by MS neurologists rather than general neurologists. Even if the objective is not to enrol in a trial, more information or a second opinion can be sought from such specialized centres.

Further reading

Polman CH, Reingold SC, Banwell B, *et al.* (2011) Diagnostic criteria for multiple sclerosis: 2010 revisions to the McDonald criteria. *Ann Neurol* **69**: 292–302.

3

Who gets MS?

➔ Key Points

- People living in moderate climates are much more likely to get MS than those living in tropical areas. Lack of sunlight is an important factor that increases the MS risk.
- When people migrate to a country with a different MS risk, the MS risk can change quite substantially, especially for young people.
- Infections do not cause MS, but do influence the risk for MS. Having had the first encounter with one particular virus relatively late in life increases the MS risk.

The World Health Organization estimates that there are around two million people worldwide that have MS. Most people who are diagnosed with MS are between 20–40 years old. MS in children is rare, but it does occur. Over the past decade, more and more research has been devoted to children with MS. Still, the vast majority of people struck by MS are young adults. Yet, MS is clearly not something that everyone on the planet is equally likely to get. The first major distinction is between men and women. Women are up to four times more likely to develop MS. This gender difference has increased over recent years. Why this is so, or why women are more likely to get MS to begin with, is not fully understood. Smoking also increases the MS risk, by about 50%. Several factors act together in causing MS. Some are linked to our genes, but quite a few other factors are part of our environment. This chapter is about the environmental factors which influence the risk of developing MS. The next chapter deals with inheritance.

It has long been obvious that the risk for MS differs substantially between different areas of the world. Most people with MS live in moderate climates in Europe, North America, Australia, and New Zealand. MS is relatively uncommon in tropical or subtropical areas, in Asia, South America, and Africa. In high-risk areas such as Scotland, as many as 2 per 1000 people have MS. For Caucasians in low-risk countries such as South Africa, this is almost 10 times less. One reason for the differences may be genes. While humans are very similar, there are genetic differences amongst races which influence the way we deal with infections, for example. Genes help determine how often we develop certain diseases, and how old we become. People of northern European descent are more likely to develop MS, a fact which is quite possibly related to special genes that only they have. Still, there are striking exceptions to this apparent link. Sami people in northern Scandinavia, for example, seem to carry certain genes which may make them relatively resistant to MS. While other people in the same area experience MS quite frequently, Sami people do so much less.

Yet, genetic differences are not enough to fully explain why MS is unevenly distributed over the world. Other factors are important too, as is apparent from the development of MS in people that have migrated to countries with an MS risk that is different from their home country. The first generation of migrants retain their genes, and probably even most of their eating habits, but start to live in a very different environment. This clearly has an impact on MS.

Does migration influence the risk of MS?

A comparison between the frequency of MS in migrants with the average MS risk in either their new country, or their country of origin, is quite revealing. Adult migrants from low-risk zones such as the Caribbean, who move to high-risk zones such as the UK, retain the same low MS risk they had at home. This is not due to some protective factor in their genes because their children, who carry the same genes, do experience a change. As they grow up in their new country, these children develop MS at similar frequencies as their new friends. When migrating before turning 15, children develop an MS risk which is higher than that of their parents, and similar to that of all the other people in their new environment. Migration from low-risk to high-risk areas is illustrated in Fig. 3.1. When people migrate the other way around, from a high-risk zone to a low-risk zone, things are different. In this case, both children and adults tend to acquire a lower MS risk, but generally not quite as low as the average for people in their new country. Especially when moving from low-risk to high-risk areas, therefore, changing countries before the age of about 15 is different from moving in adulthood.

This is quite remarkable. On average MS starts to manifest itself between the ages of 25–35. Children who develop MS are rare, as are people over the age of 50. So what happens during those first 15 years of life that influences the risk for something that becomes apparent only years later? What makes children moving to a high-risk area acquire a higher MS risk, while their parents do not? Interestingly, the two major environmental factors that we know influence MS do so most prominently in the first 15 years of life. Those two

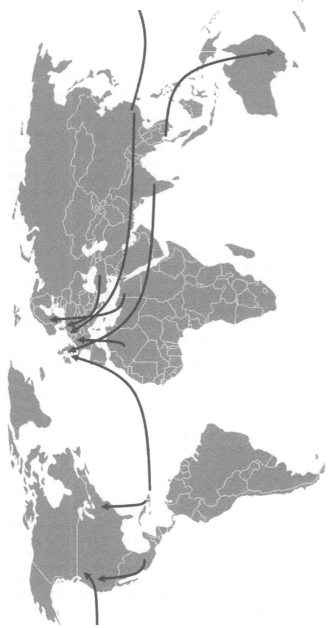

Fig. 3.1 Migration can affect the risk of developing MS. Especially for young people, moving from subtropical areas to colder and darker places increases the risk for MS.

factors are sunlight, and a certain type of infection. Let us take a closer look at them.

Sunlight and MS

There is overwhelming evidence that sunlight protects against MS, and especially so when people are young. While sunlight does several different things to our bodies, one of the most prominent things it does is to induce vitamin D production in our skin. It is very likely that this is the main reason that sunlight has its protective effect on MS. Our bodies do not produce vitamin D without sunlight. Taking vitamin D in through food is another option to boost levels, of course, but only very few types of food contain meaningful amounts of it. Unless a person takes vitamin D supplements, sunlight is by far the most important source of vitamin D. Sunlight has a marked impact on the risk for MS.

The high-risk zones for MS are all countries with a moderate climate, and moderate to low levels of sunlight. Especially in winter, the intensity of the sun in these areas is so low, that it generally fails to induce any vitamin D at all. Probably as a result of this, the further north one goes, the more frequent MS generally becomes. This has been well established in Europe and America. In the southern hemisphere, it is the other way around. People living in southern parts of Australia have a much higher risk for MS than people living in the sunny subtropical north. People on sunny mountain tops in Switzerland have MS less frequently than their countrymen in the valleys. People living in the sunnier parts of France do so too, relative to French people living in cloudier areas. Children playing outdoors in the sun develop MS much less often as compared to children who mostly stay indoors. The differences are quite substantial, and all data confirm a protective effect of sunlight and the vitamin D it induces. Adult white people with healthy levels of vitamin D have a significantly lower MS risk as compared to those with low levels of vitamin D. For children under the age of 20, the difference appears to be even larger. We will return to this subject in the chapter on non-conventional therapies (Chapter 8).

Infections and MS

Before explaining the role of infections in MS risk, we would first like to address the more basic question of whether or not MS is contagious. This question has been repeatedly raised in the past, and is not an entirely unreasonable one. Since MS was first described, and drawings were published on what MS looks like under the microscope, many people were convinced it was an infection, since it looks very much like many other brain infections. The idea that infections could cause MS was further fuelled by persistent anecdotal reports suggesting that MS would be contagious in one way or another.

One of those stories suggested that after World War II, the incidence of MS had sharply risen in the Faroe Islands. Over the period of 1943–1973, a total of 32 new cases were diagnosed, while MS was believed to have been absent from the islands in the years before. Invasion of the islands by British forces during the war were seen as the cause. Many were convinced that some MS-causing infection must have been carried to the island by the troops, or even by their dogs. How else to explain this sudden increase in MS? Because MS lesions look very much like infections, and because of a variety of such anecdotes, the belief that MS is caused by an infection has persisted. Indeed, several claims have been made over the years that an MS-specific virus or bacterium was identified. It led to newspaper reports on such exciting findings, and recommendations on how to avoid the dreaded micro-organism. However, these claims have never stood the test of time, and they are currently no longer taken seriously. There is most likely no such thing as an MS-specific virus or bacterium which directly causes the condition. Therefore, the story about the Faroe Islands and, in fact, several other anecdotes about local 'outbreaks' of MS probably reflect purely coincidental events, or may be based on incomplete information. There is compelling evidence that family members of people with MS never get 'infected' with it. We are pretty sure here. MS is not contagious.

That MS is not contagious does not mean that viruses or bacteria play no role at all. Indeed, it is quite clear that a certain virus does influence the risk for MS. Still, it could not possibly cause MS. We know this because the virus can be found in more than 90% of all adults worldwide, regardless of whether they have MS or not. The virus we are talking about is Epstein–Barr virus, or EBV, and its role in MS is a bit of a puzzle still. The most striking piece of evidence that EBV has something to do with MS is the fact that anyone who has never been infected with EBV, is highly unlikely to ever develop MS. It is almost as if the virus is required for MS to develop.

Intriguingly, age plays an important role in the effects of EBV on MS. EBV is a very common virus, spreading via saliva, and many of us run into the virus for the first time as a child, when we start to put all sorts of things into our mouth. An image of the virus is shown in Fig. 3.2. When EBV enters the body, an immune response is produced. Yet, EBV is a clever virus and despite this immune response, the virus manages to stay in our bodies for life. Usually, this causes no problems and most of the time, this is perfectly fine. However, when someone encounters EBV for the first time relatively late in life, at the age of 17 or so while kissing their first boyfriend or girlfriend, the immune response becomes different. At that age, it tends to become markedly stronger and in some cases this leads to glandular fever. Clinicians call it 'infectious mononucleosis'. In this condition, the exaggerated immune response against EBV causes extreme tiredness. While some young children also develop glandular fever, it is much more common among young adults of 15–20 years of age. Curiously, people who have experienced an episode of glandular fever have a more than twofold higher risk for MS than others. No other common infection is linked to MS in a similar way.

EBV and MS: an example of the hygiene hypothesis?

It appears that people with MS have a different relationship with EBV than others. Their immune response to EBV is different partly because they have encountered the virus for the first time at a relatively late age. It is well known that the infection rate of EBV is different in different parts of the world. In some countries such as China, almost everyone at the age of 6 has already been infected. In Scandinavia, on the other hand, more than half the children at this age are still EBV free. Exactly where we frequently find MS, people tend to experience the first EBV infection at a relatively late age. One obvious factor which contributes to this difference is the standard of healthcare. The higher this standard, the more likely it is that children remain free of infections, including with EBV, for a longer period of time. Nevertheless, with a very common virus such as EBV, even excellent healthcare standards will only delay infection, but not prevent it altogether. Thus, having an EBV

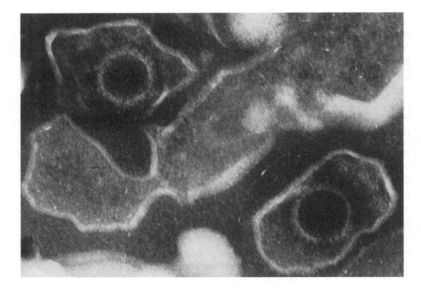

Fig. 3.2 Under a very strong microscope, two Epstein–Barr viruses become visible, along with the round cores of the virus that carries its genetic material. (Reprinted from Liza Gross et al. (2005) Virus proteins prevent cell suicide long enough to establish latent infection. *PLoS Biol* 3(12): e430, doi:10.1371/journal.pbio.0030430.)

infection early in life is associated with a low risk for MS, having it late in life is associated with a high risk.

Environmental effects and migrant data

Knowing that the most important environmental factors in MS are probably sunlight and the timing of an EBV infection, the information on the MS risk in migrants begins to make sense. To summarize again, when children up to 15 years of age move from a low-risk to a high-risk environment, they tend to acquire the high MS risk. This is different from their parents, who retain the low risk. Moving from a high-risk area to a low risk area, lowers the risk for children and their parents to some degree, but does not reduce it to the low levels seen for the native population. This is understandable if we assume that a low-risk area generally is an environment where the sun shines more brightly, and EBV infections occur at an earlier age than in a high-risk area. This is a reasonable assumption. When children grow up in a low-risk zone, they tend to be exposed to healthy doses of sunlight, and become infected with EBV relatively early in life. Both childhood factors lower the risk for MS, and this effect lasts for life. Once grown up, people who move from a low-risk to a high-risk area will therefore retain their low MS risk, the way it was established in childhood. Moving to a high-risk area when children are still young, however, changes both factors. After they have moved, sunlight exposure will go down, and the chances of rapidly becoming infected with EBV—if they haven't already—do too. Their new environment is cloudier and cleaner. The younger they move, the more these changes may increase a child's risk for MS, eventually increasing it to the level which is normal for their new country.

When people migrate the other way around, the impact is different. Sunlight conditions will often greatly improve, but it appears unlikely that Western people moving to tropical areas, for example, will start lowering their standards of hygiene. More typically, they will continue to live under housing conditions they did at home, and continue to behave in the old ways. The influence of the sun may therefore change, but the timing of EBV infections is less likely to change. Assuming that both children and adults will take advantage of higher levels of sunlight exposure, a certain decrease in the MS risk for both is quite understandable, but the change is not complete since the EBV factor will probably remain the way it was.

So what does this mean for people that already have MS?

The information on environmental factors identifies risk factors in MS, and helps us understand what may cause the disease. More importantly, it also suggests ways to prevent MS from developing as frequently as it does today. Exposing children to healthy levels of sunlight and giving them vitamin D supplements in winter will very likely help reduce future numbers of people with MS. With regard to the infectious factor, things are more complicated. It is obviously difficult to recommend lowering our hygienic standards as a preventive measure for MS. It will certainly generate quite a few other issues. Generally, one might say that one should perhaps not be too paranoid about children sharing the toys they suck on, and give them regular hugs and kisses. As a parent, you are likely to be an excellent source of an early EBV infection.

Another issue is what this means to people that have already developed MS With regard to EBV, things are simple. Essentially everyone with MS has already had their EBV infection, and there is nothing one can do to change that. Sunlight exposure and vitamin D are far more interesting. While migrant data already indicate that sunlight exposure reduces the MS risk, more recent studies suggest that sunlight and vitamin D even impact on the condition when it has already developed. In a recent study conducted in Australia, it was found that vitamin D levels in blood directly influence the risk of getting another MS relapse. The higher the levels of vitamin D, the lower the relapse risk becomes. Importantly, most of the people participating in this study did already take MS drugs. Vitamin D therefore provides an added protective effect, irrespective of whether one already takes MS drugs or not. In Chapter 8 on non-conventional therapies, we will come back to this important issue.

Further reading

Ascherio A and Munger KL (2007) Environmental risk factors for multiple sclerosis. Part I: the role of infection. *Ann Neurol* **61**: 288–99.

Ascherio A and Munger KL (2007) Environmental risk factors for multiple sclerosis. Part II: noninfectious factors. *Ann Neurol* **61**: 504–13.

Ebers GC (2008) Environmental factors and multiple sclerosis. *Lancet Neurol* 7: 268–77.

Salvetti M, Giovannoni G, and Aloisi F (2009) Epstein-Barr virus and multiple sclerosis. *Curr Opin Neurol* **22**: 201–6.

Simpson S Jr, Taylor B, Blizzard L, *et al.* (2010) Higher 25-hydroxyvitamin D is associated with lower relapse risk in multiple sclerosis. *Ann Neurol* **68**: 193–203.

Zaadstra BM, Chorus AM, van Buuren S, *et al.* (2008) Selective association of multiple sclerosis with infectious mononucleosis. *Mult Scler* **14**: 307–13.

4

Is MS hereditary?

> ### → Key Points
>
> - MS is not directly inherited.
> - Genes impact on the risk of developing MS, but apart from identical twins, even the closest relatives of someone with MS have a more than 95% chance of never developing MS themselves.
> - The impact of genes on MS is complicated, and influenced by the environment. Place and date of birth therefore influence the genetic risk.

We are familiar with the idea that certain diseases run in some families. This is because many diseases develop at least partly due to 'bad' genes. If a person has a disease caused by such genes, others in the family are more likely than average to get the disease too, since they share some of their genes. In this context, identical twins are interesting since they share all their genes. The more often identical twins develop the same rare disease, the stronger the hereditary factor probably is. When one identical twin develops MS, the chance that the other does so too is much higher than average, between 15–35%. For anyone else, it is around 0.1%. As identical twins therefore show us, sharing all genes with someone that has developed MS strongly increases the risk for MS. A hereditary factor in MS clearly exists. Still, the risk for identical twins is far from 100%, clarifying that MS is not determined by genes alone. In this chapter, we will explain more on the nature of the hereditary factor, and summarize information on the risks for family members of people with MS.

Genes and DNA

To appreciate what risk genes in MS actually mean, it is useful to first clarify something about genes and inheritance. Not all of us have had full training in genetics. What is a gene anyway? In the human body, there are an almost endless number of substances that we need for survival. Almost all of them have to be made inside of our bodies, since food does not supply them. After all, we are no cannibals. One group of substances in our body is called 'proteins', some of which are also known as 'enzymes'. Proteins are a crucial part of the collection of the body's substances, since they take care of making pretty much all other substances, including fats and sugars, and other proteins again. By and large, the body can be run perfectly well only by making sure that the right proteins are there, since they will then take care of the rest. Each protein is unique, and produced according to very specific building instructions. The instructions to build a single protein are called genes. A gene is a segment of DNA in which the different chemical building blocks that make up DNA are strung together in a specific order (see Fig. 4.1). Just like letters form words, the order of the building blocks in a gene forms the building instructions for a particular protein. It is currently estimated that humans have about 23,000 different genes. All those genes are packed together into long strings of DNA, called chromosomes. These, in turn, are wrapped up inside the core of cells.

Inheriting genes and traits

Most people are probably more interested in traits than in genes. The term 'trait' means the visible manifestation of our genes, such as having blue eyes, being tall, or, indeed, carrying a certain risk to develop MS. Simple traits rely on only a few genes, but inheriting the tendency to develop a certain chronic disease is usually more complicated. It is important to appreciate that traits are inherited in a different way from genes. Let's first look at genes.

As explained earlier, all our genes are contained in separate segments of DNA. Long strings of these are called chromosomes. We have two sets of 23 such chromosomes in almost every cell of our body. In each reproductive cell, however, we only have one set of them. When the reproductive cells of two partners successfully combine, the new fertilized cell that is created contains a full duplicate set of genes again, one from each partner. This is the start of

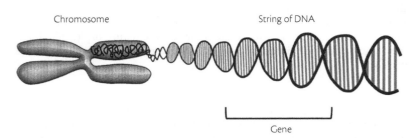

Fig. 4.1 A gene is a segment of the DNA string with its double helix, which makes up our chromosomes. Every gene is a recipe for a certain protein. The order of the chemicals in the DNA string encodes this recipe.

a new individual. Our next child relies on us doing it again, but each time it happens, the genes are reshuffled before being passed on. After all, our reproductive cells may carry either of the two sets of genes we have, and there is no reason to pass on the same one every time.

As the result of each parent contributing half their genes to offspring, children share half their genes with each of their parents. They also share half their genes with each brother or sister, but the shared portion is different every time. Brothers and sisters can be quite alike, but strikingly different too. This also applies to non-identical twins. Genetically speaking, they are no different from any other brother or sister. They just happened to be born at the same time. Identical twins are a special case. They share all their genes, since they both emerged from a single fertilized cell, as shown in Fig. 4.2. As the family relationship weakens, the percentage of genes that are shared goes down. For example, we share 25% of our genes with any of our grandparents, and 12.5% with our cousins. Thus, every reproduction step that separates family members reduces the shared portion of genes by 50%. How this affects inheritance of 'bad' genes that predispose to a disease, is illustrated in Fig. 4.3.

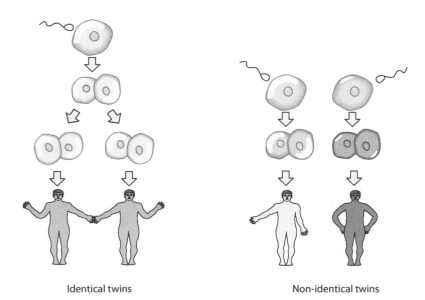

Identical twins   Non-identical twins

Fig. 4.2 The chance that the identical twin of someone with MS also develops MS, is much higher than that for a non-identical twin. This observation held the key to a much better understanding of the inheritance of MS.

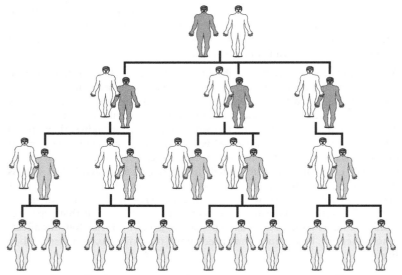

Fig. 4.3 If a set of 'bad' genes increases the risk to develop a disease, the effect may be watered down by 'healthy' genes from the partners. While being passed on to next generations, 'bad' and 'healthy' genes are mixed in every round of reproduction. Only if a single 'bad' gene is dominant, will its effects persist in the family members who have inherited that gene.

Inheriting traits

Inheriting traits is different from inheriting genes, for a number of reasons. First, visible traits tend to result from different genes acting together. Very often, the final result is not just the sum of what each individual gene does, but a very different one. This is because genes influence each other. They may block each other's effects, they may reinforce them, or produce an intermediate outcome. Mixing genes for blue eyes with those for brown eyes may well lead to green eyes.

Secondly, there is also another phenomenon that makes traits dependent on more than genes alone. Researchers call it 'epigenetic regulation'. Don't worry about this difficult term. You already know exactly what it is, although you may never have realized it is called this. It turns your hair grey as you grow old. Try a mirror. The grey hairs you may see are not the worn down hairs you had when you were 10 years old. They are new hairs that one fine day started to come out grey. For some reason, the substance that gave your hair its original colour when you were young has stopped appearing. This is the result of 'epigenetic regulation'. It means that changes associated with age have made the hair colour gene in the string of DNA inaccessible to the hair-producing machinery. You still have the gene, but it is no longer possible for the machinery that produces hair to consult it.

Also for other reasons, having a certain gene is no guarantee that it is used all the time, or even used at all. It is a bit like having recipes. In your own cookery books in the kitchen, you may have the recipe for boeuf bourguignon somewhere. Yet, you are unlikely to prepare it every single day. Your body also does not read all its genetic recipes every day. In addition, since the impact of a gene is often influenced by other genes, inheriting a certain gene does not necessarily mean that it has the same effect in your body as it has in someone else's. In your kitchen, boeuf bourguignon may come out slightly differently from Jamie Oliver's kitchen. All these effects influence the final translation of genes into traits. Traits are therefore inherited in much more complicated and subtle ways than genes, and their manifestations are influenced by age and environment. This is a crucial aspect of inheritance of traits to keep in mind, and it turns out to be very important for understanding the inheritance of MS.

Inheriting MS: many different genes?

How the risk of developing MS is passed on to the next generation is still the subject of research today. Much has already been clarified, but a few things are still not clear. To understand the inheritance of MS, it is crucial to understand the data that have been collected on twins. As we said before, the MS risk for someone whose identical twin brother or sister has MS is much higher than that of an average person. In Canada, for example, it is about 200 times higher than average, at 35%. The risk for a non-identical twin is much lower, about 3.5%. This is actually quite strange. Identical twins share 100% of their genes, while non-identical twins share 50% of them, which is only two times less. Why is their MS risk ten times lower than that of an identical twin, and not simply two times lower?

For a long time, this curious difference was explained by assuming that the MS risk is not determined by a single gene, but by the cooperation of different MS genes. The idea was that these MS genes would work together to create a final risk, like football players work together towards a common goal. If all these genes would reinforce each other's individual minor contribution to the risk for MS, together they would create a major 'team effect', explaining the unusually strong genetic effect in identical twins.

Today, however, thinking about MS genes has started to go in another direction. The new idea is that there is, in fact, only a single gene which largely determines the risk for MS, but that environmental factors strongly influence the way this gene works. In other words, there is good evidence that there are not many different genes working together to create a strong MS link between identical twins, but a single gene working together with the environment. Importantly, the environmental factors already start to influence the risk for MS before birth.

Inheriting MS: genes and environment work together

One reason for the change in thinking has been new data on the frequency at which identical twins both have MS. This frequency is called 'the concordance rate'. The first large-scale studies on this issue were performed in Canada. These studies revealed that the Canadian concordance rate is about 35%. Surprisingly, the concordance rate in Italy is only about 15%, more than two times less than in Canada. This is quite remarkable since identical twins in Italy obviously share the same 100% of their genes as twins do in Canada. So what causes the difference? One way to explain it would be to assume that the environment makes a difference. It is obvious that sunlight exposure and feeding habits in Italy, for example, are quite different from Canada. As explained earlier, such factors can change the impact of genes, and therefore, could conceivably also change their impact on the MS risk. But is there any evidence that the environment can do this?

The answer is yes. Recent data have revealed that the month of birth makes a difference for the risk for MS. In the northern hemisphere, people have a slightly higher chance to develop MS when born in May or June, while people have a slightly lower chance when born around November. In the southern hemisphere, it is the other way around. Australian people born in November have a higher MS risk. Only the sun can explain this. When a mother is exposed to healthy doses of sunlight during pregnancy in the summer, the chance of developing MS for her children subsequently born in autumn is reduced. A pregnancy during winter, on the other hand, when sunlight is scarce, generates a higher risk for the child. Clearly, it already matters under which conditions the mother lives through pregnancy.

So what makes identical twins different from other family members? Currently, it is believed that the interplay between environment and genes can explain the difference. Identical twins not only share all their genes, but also the time of birth. The conditions under which they spent the first part of their lives, including the time prior to birth, are exactly the same. They shared nutrients they received from their mother, and shared the same blood levels of vitamin D, for example. While non-identical twins are obviously also born at the same time, they do not share all their genes, but only half of them. In non-identical twins, therefore, the environmental effects around birth cannot act on the same set of genes. Therefore, being born at the same time does not produce the same long-term effects in non-identical twins as it does in identical twins. For this reason, non-identical twins do not share the high concordance rates seen in identical twins. They just share the risk that all brothers and sisters share.

So which gene is now important?

For many years, it has been known that one particular gene is very important for the inherited risk for MS. As explained earlier, recent data now indicate that only this gene really matters. Other genes have rather small additional effects at best. After a long search for other MS genes, we have therefore now returned to the one gene that was known all along. This gene is called the 'major histocompatibility complex' or 'MHC' for short. The protein this gene encodes is aptly called 'MHC protein'. A little more of what MHC proteins do, is explained in the chapter that deals with the immune system. MHC proteins are crucial for our ability to mount immune responses, including those that cause tissue rejection after organ transplantations. The term 'histo-compatibility' (meaning tissue compatibility) refers to this particular effect. Since MHC genes exist in dozens of different versions among humans, and since few tolerate each other, organ transplantation works best when MHC proteins from the donor and the recipient are very similar. The recipient will otherwise reject the transplant. MHC protein variants control immune responses, and can instruct such a response to be aggressive, mild, or something in between. It is therefore no surprise that the MHC gene influences the risk for MS in different ways, dependent on which of the variant MHC proteins are present. Some of them increase the MS risk, while others reduce the risk. The effect can be as strong as a factor of four to six either way. Which effects on the MS risk are caused by the many different MHC gene variants are now being studied in more detail.

Recently, it has become clear that, in rare cases, another gene may play an important role as well, and can actually cause MS. This gene, called CYP27B1 encodes an enzyme that helps generate the biologically active form of vitamin D. If there is something wrong with this gene in such a way that vitamin D levels in the body are strongly reduced, MS will also develop. This is a special and very rare case, however, which probably helps explain no more than 1 in every 500 MS cases. It does, however, emphasize the importance of vitamin D, as discussed further on in this book.

The bottom line

The inheritance of MS is not just about genes. Except perhaps for some rare cases, as discussed previously, it is generally impossible to examine someone's DNA profile, and predict whether they will develop MS or not. Even when one carries the worst possible MHC genes, the chance to never develop MS is

Table 4.1 Approximate MS risks for family members of people with MS in the UK.

Family bond	MS risk (%)
Father	2.0
Mother	2.0
Brother	3.2
Identical twin	25.0
Sister	4.4
Son	0.6
Daughter	3.2
Nephew	1.0
Niece	2.3
Paternal uncle	0.8
Paternal aunt	1.2
Maternal uncle	0.7
Maternal aunt	0.8
First cousin	0.9

Source: data from Alastair Compston and Alasdair Coles, Multiple sclerosis, *The Lancet*, Volume **372**, Issue 9648, 25–31 October 2008, Pages 1502–17, copyright Elsevier.

still more than 99%. In addition, the effect of the most important MS gene is strongly influenced by the environment. The two factors work together. The MS risk for family members of someone with MS therefore also depends on the environment. The concordance rate of MS in identical twins in the UK is about 25%, in Canada, it is about 35%, and in Italy about 15%. The risk that MS is passed from mother to children additionally depends on the time of the year the mother is pregnant. Being pregnant in winter makes mothers more likely to pass on MS. It also matters whether the mother ate fatty fish during pregnancy since this reduces the risk. In other words, Table 4.1 which lists the average risks for family members in the UK, inevitably falls short in providing exact risks that are applicable to everyone. The numbers will vary from one country to the next, and they are influenced by the several different other factors we have now clarified.

New data on MS genes other than the MHC gene are of interest to research-ers, as they point out which proteins are relevant to the development of MS, at least to some extent. Most of these appear to be involved in controlling our immune system. Yet, the effect of each of these genes on the overall genetic risk for MS is very small indeed. For people that carry such genes, they there-fore make rather little difference in real life. From a genetic point of view, family members of people with MS need not worry too much. Only for identical twins the inherited MS risk is significant when one of the twins has already developed MS. This is because only here the influence of the shared early environment in life fully kicks in because all the relevant genes are shared too. It is really an exception. Risks for any family member other than an identical twin are well below 5%. When thinking about the risks for any children, one may interpret the current data to mean that MS remains largely a case of bad luck, with all due respect to genetic researchers.

Further reading

Fugger L, Friese MA, and Bell JI (2009) From genes to function: the next challenge to understanding multiple sclerosis. *Nat Rev Immunol* **9**: 408–17.

Giovannoni G and Ebers G (2007) Multiple sclerosis: the environment and causation. *Curr Opin Neurol* **20:** 261–8.

Ramagopalan SV, Knight JC, and Ebers GC (2009) Multiple sclerosis and the major histocompatibility complex. *Curr Opin Neurol* **22**: 219–25.

The International Multiple Sclerosis Genetics Consortium (2011) Genetic risk and a primary role for cell-mediated immune mechanisms in multiple sclerosis. *Nature* **476**: 214–19.

5

What causes MS? Meet the immune system

⊃ Key Points

 ◆ The immune system is made up of many, very mobile cells that continuously move around, communicate, and produce many different substances.

 ◆ Immune cells eliminate invading micro-organisms and emerging tumours. However, not all immune responses are destructive. The immune system also actively switches itself off, and starts repair of damaged tissue.

 ◆ By and large, the immune system knows which substances belong to the body, and which do not. In addition, it distinguishes dangerous substances from harmless ones. Harmless substances are not attacked, even when they are strange.

When considering what might cause MS, the immune system immediately attracts our attention. Inspection of MS lesions under the microscope makes it clear that immune cells destroy the tissue. We know that antibodies, unmistakable signs of immune responses, are present in brain and spinal cord fluid of people with MS. This is still used as one of the diagnostic criteria. The gene that impacts most on the risk for MS, the MHC gene, regulates immune responses. Most of the other genes with a minor impact on MS do too. Blocking the immune system, like modern drugs do, slows down the disease. Also, there are animal models that are used to mimic MS. In these models, activation of the animal's immune system with proteins from the brain or spinal cord causes destructive lesions similar to MS. Clearly, any discussion about what might cause MS must involve the immune system. Unfortunately, the immune system is complicated. Explaining it in the context of this book truly is a daunting task. We have therefore limited things to what we consider the most relevant aspects of the immune system, and conveniently ignore many details.

The immune system, a bird's eye view

Even Wikipedia gets overwhelmed when it comes to the immune system. On its website, it defines the immune system as 'a system of biological structures and processes within an organism that protects against disease by identifying and killing pathogens and tumour cells'. This is similar to what most textbooks would say, and this certainly describes an important part of it. Yet, this only describes half the immune system's job. The other half is to ensure that once started, immune reactions are shut down again, and that any damage to organs or tissues is repaired. In addition, the immune system is continuously trying to prevent any useless or dangerous immune response from starting in the first place. Not having an immune response or shutting it down often takes as much effort as having one.

So what is this 'system of biological structures and processes'? Probably the best way to understand it is to think in terms of individual cells, the surface of these cells, and the chemicals they produce. Cells of the immune system are everywhere in our body. Some reside in special organs, such as spleen, thymus, or lymph nodes, and many float around in our blood, as illustrated in Fig. 5.1. All of them, however, are surprisingly mobile. Continuous movement of these cells is a fundamental trait of the immune system. It allows immune cells to monitor our entire body and to rapidly communicate with each other. They do so by touching each other's surface, and by smelling each other's secreted chemicals. Such contacts can make immune cells divide, produce new substances, and move into tissues. They can even tell each other to die, but despite this, it is quite a lively set of cells.

The innate and adaptive immune system

Cells of the immune system are divided into two groups. One group is called the innate immune system. From the day they are formed, these cells rapidly respond to anything they regard as dangerous or strange. On their surface, innate immune cells carry a range of antennas, or 'receptors' as immunologists call them, to sense the presence of bacteria, viruses, or dying cells. These antennas on innate cells are not very discriminating. The substances they sense are usually things that many bacteria or viruses have in common. When these antennas register the presence of something which does not belong in the body, innate immune cells respond rapidly, often within just minutes. Macrophages, for example, are such cells. They reside in many parts of our body, and can be regarded as our first line of defence as well as the garbage removal service. Immediately upon contact with something they dislike, they engulf and destroy it. In this way, innate immune cells can deal with bacteria, viruses, dead cells, inhaled dust particles, wood or glass splinters, anything that they regard as not being useful or potentially dangerous.

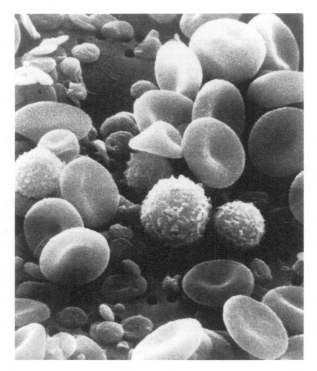

Fig. 5.1 The immune system is a collection of cells which act together to fight off infections and tumours. They also make sure that immune reactions are stopped, and damaged tissue is repaired. This image shows these immune cells in blood (Photograph by Bruce Wetzel and Harry Schaefer. Reproduced with permission of National Cancer Institute.).

A crucial feature of innate cells is that they repeat their same defensive actions over and over again.

The second group of immune cells are called the adaptive (or acquired) immune system. They are cells that don't immediately respond like innate cells but take care of the follow-up. In contrast to innate immune cells, they are very picky indeed. This is because each of them has an antenna which senses only a single small fragment of a single bacterium, virus, or tumour cell. While there are several different types of adaptive immune cells, the most important ones are what we call 'T cells', white blood cells that always pass through the thymus when they mature, hence the 'T'. We will use T cells as an example of adaptive immune cells.

The specificity of immune reactions

T cells only come into action after their antenna has sensed the presence of a bacterial or viral fragment on the surface of an innate immune cell such as a macrophage, as illustrated in Fig. 5.2. We call such microbial fragments 'antigens'. The proteins on the macrophage surface that displays these antigens are called MHC proteins. They have already been mentioned in the chapter on genes and inheritance. The T-cell antenna cannot sense any free-floating antigens, but is fully dependent on the macrophage first displaying them on its surface using these MHC proteins. Each T cell carries only one type of antenna for this purpose, and the antenna is very picky indeed. When a macrophage that has engulfed a bacterium or virus meets up with T cells, only the few T cells with an antenna that precisely fits any of the antigens on MHC proteins displayed by macrophages will respond. Other T cells will not be bothered.

T cells with the right antenna will first start to multiply. This is because we only have a few T cells for each of the many different antigens, and we need many more of them to mount a successful immune attack. The resulting population of daughter cells all inherit the exact same antenna, and respond to the exact same antigen as the mother cell did. This ability to recognize that

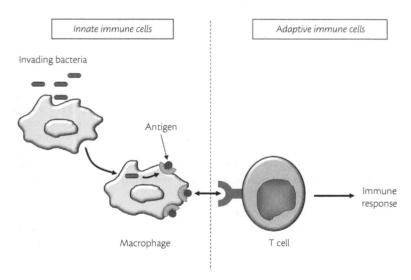

Fig. 5.2 After innate cells have cleared invading bacteria, they display fragments of those bacteria (antigens) on their surface. MHC proteins are used for this display. Cells of the adaptive immune system, such as T cells, may or may not recognize those displayed fragments. If they do, they may start an immune response.

particular antigen and no other, is what we call 'antigenic specificity' or pickiness. After 1 or 2 weeks, there are enough daughter cells to deal with the invader in a more sophisticated manner. These daughter cells ensure that even cells in which the invader may be hiding, are killed. They also make sure that other immune cells, called B cells, will start to produce antibodies with a precisely matching antigenic specificity. Such antibodies can stick to the bacteria, viruses, or tumour cells that carried the original antigen, making it much easier for macrophages to track them down, and kill them.

After the damage has been cleared, a few of the daughter T cells as well as some of the antibodies remain, and persist for many years. As a result, this part of the immune system can strike back much faster the second time it is confronted with the same invader. This is why we call this the 'adaptive' immune system. Its cells have adapted to the original invader, and they remember that it needs to be attacked. It is the basis of specific immunological memory, a state we refer to as 'being immune'. The antigenic specificity of T cells and antibodies make them very effective against one particular invader, but not against any other one. If another virus or bacterium comes along, from which new and different antigens will be generated and displayed by macrophages, the adaptive immune system has to start all over again. This is why we are not immune to a newly emerging flu virus, despite having built up an immune response against earlier versions. When a new virus yields different antigens, our immune system sees it as a different thing altogether.

Immunological tolerance

Cells of the immune system have a way to decide whether or not it is useful to mount a defensive response against something they encounter. In a healthy body, the very mobile immune cells continuously bump into things. As a rule, they are not bothered by that. This is just as well, since the body's own normal substances obviously do not require an immune attack. This state of immune cells not being bothered by something they bump into, is called 'immunological tolerance'. At school, we were taught that immunological tolerance is the result of the immune system distinguishing 'self' from 'foreign' substances. This is only part of the story.

Immunological tolerance is controlled by several mechanisms. The mechanism they were talking about at school is called 'central tolerance'. It means that newly formed T cells trying to leave the thymus are subjected to a test. This test includes offering them substances that are present in the thymus. If a newly formed T cell responds to any of the substances on display, it fails the test and is killed. The thymus is rather unforgiving. Just as well, because whatever was on display in the thymus clearly belongs to the body, and requires no attack. Indeed, central tolerance makes sure that the immune system avoids responding to at least some 'self' substances.

However, there are substances in our body that are not present in the thymus. The mechanism of central tolerance is therefore not suited to kill T cells that react to substances that may be present elsewhere in the body. To control T cells that may react to such substances, the immune system uses additional 'on' and 'off' signals. This level of control is called 'peripheral tolerance'. When T cells encounter something they recognize, accompanying 'off' signals will still prevent them from responding. Sometimes, it even tells the T cells to actively switch off any response that might have already started. Importantly, when giving these 'on' or 'off' signals, the immune system does not make a distinction between 'self' or 'foreign', but between 'harmless' and 'dangerous'. There is a very good reason for choosing this basis for deciding on whether or not to mount an immune attack. There are simply too many 'foreign' substances in our body to attack. Think of all the food we eat. All of it is 'foreign' but, none of it requires an immune attack. Most of the 'foreign' substances in our body are actually essential for our well-being. Our gastrointestinal tract, for example, is filled with billions of harmless bacteria that help digest food, and keep other, more dangerous bacteria away from our body. Many of these gut bacteria are actually sold as probiotic supplements, advertised as being helpful to our immune system.

Obviously we need to allow 'foreign' food substances into our body, along with beneficial 'foreign' microbes. For this reason, our immune system cannot rely on distinguishing 'foreign' from 'self'. So it does not. Instead, it distinguishes 'dangerous' from 'harmless' by examining whether or not there is any damage around. Cells of the innate system are the ones to register such damage, and they make an initial decision whether something is harmless or dangerous. Macrophages, for example, raise the alarm and switch to 'on' when they sense something dangerous. When that happens, they stimulate a response by T cells against anything of interest they might find in the area. When there is no damage, macrophages remain calm and give the 'off' signal. In this case, anything in the area will be tolerated by T cells, even clearly foreign bacteria and viruses. Obviously, the immune system is flexible and while the described principles govern it, terms and conditions apply. The 'off' sign of macrophages, for example, may turn into an 'on' sign when their decision that a substance is harmless, is overruled by pre-existing immunity against that substance. More about this flexibility is explained later.

The colour codes of the immune system

So far, we have described the activities of innate and adaptive immune cells, using macrophages and T cells as examples, in a black-and-white manner. We have explained what turns them on or off, as if activation of immune cells would always result in the same type of response. It is slightly more complicated than that. Immune cells come in different flavours. Rest assured, after explaining this extra complication, we will leave it at that. The reason why we bother with this complication is that some MS drugs work at this level. They change the flavours of immune cells. In general, there are three different main flavours of activation for both innate and adaptive immune cells. Intermediary forms can exist, but we will ignore these for the moment. To keep things simple we will use colour codes to distinguish them. As illustrated in Fig. 5.3, the first is a 'code red' response. It is an aggressive type of response, which unleashes the full power of the immune system to destroy whatever triggered it. The second type we will call a 'code yellow' response, and the third a 'code green'. The 'code yellow' response involves a more balanced immune response. Elements of the immune system that can be destructive are activated, but so are elements that tone it down, or even block some immune activities. In this way, a full-blown destructive response is avoided, and turned into a much milder version.

Finally, the 'code green' response makes sure the aggressive parts of immune responses are switched off altogether, and that repair processes are started. It gives the go ahead for new tissue to be formed to replace any damaged material. Thus, the variety of colour codes plays an essential role in allowing the immune system to perform a wide range of different functions, from mounting

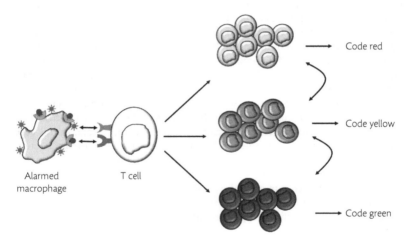

Fig. 5.3 When alarmed, the immune system not only decides whether or not it will respond to invading microbes, or any damage to tissue. It also decides how it will respond. Different 'colour codes' exist for immune responses. Responses may be aggressive and destructive (code red), they may be designed to actually stop immune responses and start repair processes (code green), or something in between (code yellow). The immune system may continuously change its colour codes, dependent on the situation.

a full-blown attack on invaders, toning down its destructive activity, to switching itself off and stimulating tissue repair once an attack has met with success. Without colour codes, we would be in trouble, as all immune responses would go on forever. This would clearly not be a great idea.

Autoimmunity: the distinction between 'self' and 'non-self'

With a clearer view of the immune system, it is time to address the issue of autoimmunity. After all, that is what MS is believed to be about. In the previous paragraphs, we have described the general way the immune system works, or rather, should work. Is autoimmunity a mistake? Is it a deviation from the rules? Or does autoimmunity exist precisely because of the rules?

When talking about autoimmunity, it is good to first remind ourselves that our immune system may not be perfect yet. Evolution is still going on. One thing that the immune system may still not be able to adequately deal with, is the fact that substances in our body are not always precisely the same. Apart from our bodies gradually changing as we get older, there are sometimes quite rapid changes in cells and tissues that the immune system may be confused by. Such changes may be brought about by an infection, for example. Quite often, the presence of a virus or bacterium inside a cell makes it suddenly produce new substances, to protect itself from the dangers arising. Exposure to a toxic chemical, or a sudden shortage of oxygen, may trigger similar effects. The newly appearing substances may be necessary to prevent the cell from dying. Unfortunately, the normal ways to secure immunological tolerance may sometimes not work so well for unexpected temporary products, despite the fact that they are part of our own bodies.

As we have explained, 'self' substances outside the thymus can still become the target of an immune response, despite being 'self'. Not having seen them in the thymus, T cells are simply not aware that such substances are 'self'. When a 'self' substance then appears in full view for the first time and is accompanied by the signs of danger, for example, in an infected cell, it may easily become the target of a specific immune response. In fact, this happens in all of us. During the many normal infections and other little mishaps that we all undergo, protective 'self' substances temporarily emerge in affected cells, and they become a target of the immune system. After all, macrophages in this context will be quite likely to raise the danger flag. Just as much as the immune system builds up immunity against viruses or bacteria in infected cells, it will build up immunity against previously unseen 'self' substances. This will lead to some level of autoimmunity building up in all of us. It is perfectly normal.

Taking the rules of the immune system into account, autoimmunity is therefore normal. Many autoimmune reactions actually help keep the immune system in check, and promote healing processes. Other, more aggressive autoimmune reactions may also not necessarily pose a problem. After all, the 'self' target will only be attacked when it is accompanied by the signs of damage. In a healthy body, this simply does not happen, and no immune cell will be bothered by the presence of 'self' target. Clearly, things change when the 'self' target resurfaces in a location where damage emerges at the same time. If it is another infection that causes this, there would still be no problem since in that case, an added immune response to a 'self' substance in the context of an infection may actually help clear that infection even more effectively. If it is a dying cell that produces it, this is fine too. Dying cells must be discarded. The real problem, and the condition that might cause an autoimmune disease, only arises if the 'self' target appears in the absence of an infection or a lethal problem for the cell, and is still accompanied by signs of damage. While this is unusual, it is clearly not impossible. This is what we probably need to look for in MS.

So is there anything wrong with the immune system during MS?

As it has now turned out, autoimmunity is not something unique to people with an autoimmune disease. It is actually quite normal, and certainly not necessarily dangerous. Questions remaining now are whether or not in people with MS, this autoimmune function is different, stronger perhaps. Also, might it be directed against somewhat different substances, the ones that can be found in our brain or spinal cord? Do any of the protective temporary substances play a role in confusing the immune system in people with MS? In the next chapter, we will summarize what researchers have found when trying to answer these questions.

Further reading

Frohman EM, Racke MK, and Raine CS (2006) Multiple sclerosis—the plaque and its pathogenesis. *New Engl J Med* **354:** 942–55.

Kono H, Rock KL (2008) How dying cells alert the immune system to danger. *Nat Rev Immunol* **8:** 279–89.

Mosser DM and Edwards JP (2008) Exploring the full spectrum of macrophage activation. *Nat Rev Immunol* **8:** 958–69.

Woodland DL and Kohlmeier JE (2009) Migration, maintenance and recall of memory T cells in peripheral tissues. *Nat Rev Immunol* **9:** 153–61.

Zhou L, Chong MM, and Littman DR (2009) Plasticity of CD4 + T-cell differentiation. *Immunity* **30:** 646–55.

6

What causes MS? Is it really the immune system?

⮕ Key Points

◆ We do not know what causes MS. Here, we discuss some ideas about possible culprits that have been suggested over the years. They include certain viruses and bacteria, toxic chemicals, amalgam fillings, or food components. Recently, obstructed blood vessels have been added to the list.

◆ The immune system is often blamed for causing MS, but this is a misunderstanding. The immune system of people with MS is normal. It is involved in the process, but it does not cause MS.

While we do not know the cause of MS, we will discuss some ideas that have been put forward. The immune system has been widely blamed for MS for one obvious reason: it is the machinery that creates an MS lesion. Some might think that the immune system is therefore the cause of MS. Case solved. Clearly, this is not very satisfactory. The next question is, of course, why the immune system shows this activity in the brain and spinal cord of people with MS and not in others. There must be something special which causes the immune system to destroy myelin and nerve fibres only in people with MS. In the previous chapter, we have introduced the immune system, and tried to explain some of its most important rules of engagement. If you missed this chapter, or found it too confusing, this is no problem. We will summarize a few things again when we need to. This chapter is understandable on its own.

People have also blamed certain viruses or bacteria for MS. Several other diseases of the brain that look like MS are caused by an infection, so it makes sense to explore the possibility that this could be the case in MS too. Food is another favourite, including, for example, dairy products, or a variety of antibiotics or hormones contained in food. Yet other potential causes have been considered, toxic chemicals, for example, such as mercury which can leak from the fillings in our teeth. More recently, restricted blood vessels have been suggested as a cause. Is there something in these claims? Since MS is more prevalent in Western societies than in less developed countries, other creative attempts have been made to examine if Western lifestyle factors might cause MS. Having had a root-canal treatment, for example, or living close to high-voltage power lines. Over the years, there have been several truly heroic attempts to explain it all.

Is MS caused by immune cells that attack myelin?

One of the most widely repeated statements on MS is that it is caused by an autoimmune attack on the myelin sheath. The picture painted is that of immune cells invading the brain and attacking myelin. If this were indeed the case, it should be possible to find something in the immune system of people with MS that is different from others. Surely, if immune cells continuously invade the brain and spinal cord, it must be possible to detect these deviant and aggressive cells in blood samples? Importantly, the immune cells should specifically target myelin and nerve fibres. After all, people with MS are not more likely to develop any other disease, allergy, or autoimmune condition. They only have inflammatory damage in the brain and spinal cord, but not in their joints, pancreas, or skin. When searching for abnormal immune activity in people with MS, researchers have therefore examined many features of immune cells hoping to find something that explains the immune attack on myelin and nerve fibres. To date, however, still no evidence has been found to indicate that the immune system in a person with MS is any different from someone else's, in a way that would explain MS. Immune cells are present that could participate in an attack on myelin, but these cells are also present in other people. Their presence, as such, is perfectly normal.

It is important to appreciate this point. Not only does it mean that we need to look away from the immune system to find the real cause of MS, it also puts current drug treatments in an interesting perspective. Current drugs for MS target the immune system. As explained later, essentially all current and emerging MS drugs are aimed at suppressing general functions of the immune system, often not in very well-defined ways. While this may indeed provide some relief, the fact that the immune system itself does not cause MS means that current treatment options in MS address the symptoms, but not the cause of the problem.

MS lesions start from within the brain itself

Declaring the immune system innocent of causing MS may create some confusion. After all, immune cells are obviously involved in destroying myelin during the inflammatory reaction that is typical for MS, once this reaction gets going. Looking at brain tissue under a microscope tells us so. When the immune cells are not the cause, why are they there, and why are they activated?

At this point we have to return to the information on immunological tolerance we discussed earlier on. Importantly, the immune system is controlled by 'on' and 'off' switches in various tissues and organs, which reflect the presence or absence of tissue damage or disturbances. Cells of the innate immune system, such as macrophages, control these switches. Because of this basic rule of engagement, the accumulation and activity of adaptive immune cells in a certain place of our body is critically dependent on the presence of tissue damage or disturbances at that site. In other words, a local event of tissue disturbance registered by a macrophage is usually the first step in an immune reaction, not a large-scale invasion by adaptive immune cells. This applies to the brain and spinal cord just as much as it applies to other tissues and organs. Thus, given that there is nothing wrong with immune cells in people with MS, maybe there is a problem within the brain and spinal cord itself, in a way that upsets macrophages?

Careful examination of brain tissue of people with MS has indeed begun to reveal the presence of mild abnormalities and disturbances, even before blood-borne cells of the adaptive immune system are there to start any trouble. The local disturbances are very subtle at an early stage, and can be seen under the microscope only when specific staining chemicals are used. We have shown them in the first chapter. Also brain scans may reveal abnormal activity. Importantly, series of such scans taken over periods of weeks or months have clarified that the local tissue abnormalities may precede the appearance of a traditional, full-blown destructive MS lesion in that location. It all seems to start right there. Research as to how local damage or disturbances in the brain and spinal cord provoke an immune attack on myelin, has only just started. It appears more than likely that the real cause of MS is to be found there. Not in our immune system as such, but in the tissue that is under attack, the central nervous system. The recurrent nature of the problem, with lesions appearing and disappearing all the time, suggests that whatever makes the local immune switch jump to 'on', is equally persistent.

In the previous chapter, we have explained how temporary protective substances that are made by cells under stress can confuse the immune system. Not having learned that these temporary substances actually belong to the body, the immune system might attack them, when it also detects signs of damage. It would attack them just as much as it would attack a virus or bacterium. Intriguingly, areas of the brains of people with MS show abnormal innate immune cell activity, even before immune cells move in from the bloodstream. In these areas, some protective substances can indeed be found in myelin-forming cells. It is known that at least one of those protective substances, called alpha B-crystallin, is a target of pre-existing immunity in humans. The appearance of this substance in cells under stress could therefore well turn out to be important as a trigger of an immune reaction. Research into this issue currently continues.

One can only speculate about the real cause for the myelin-forming cells to become distressed in people with MS, accumulate protective substances, and for neighbouring innate immune cells such as macrophages to take it as a sign of danger. One obvious possibility is, of course, that a bacterial or viral infection of myelin-forming cells generates the disturbance that is visible. Do we have any evidence that this happens?

Are infections to blame?

Although we have explained before that MS is not contagious, an infection deep in our brain and spinal cord, where the myelin-forming cells are, may not

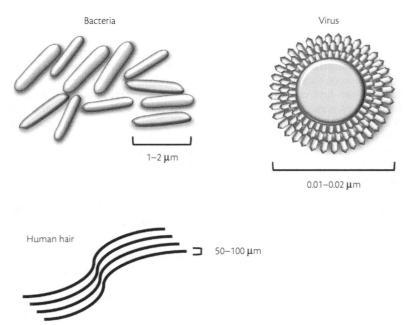

Fig. 6.1 It is not easy to see a virus or bacterium because they are very small. Here their sizes are compared to the thickness of a human hair. One μm (micrometre) is a millionth part of a metre.

necessarily be contagious. After all, for a microbe to be contagious, it must be able to get out of the central nervous system again and spread to other people. Not all microbes may necessarily be able to do that. Given this possibility, many researchers have looked for possibly relevant bacteria or viruses in people with MS, by examining brain tissue or spinal fluid for such very small creatures (see Fig. 6.1).

Despite several claims that have been made over the years, there is no evidence that brain or spinal cord tissue from people with MS is infected with a virus or bacterium which could directly cause the immune reactions of MS. Different from causing problems by directly infecting cells in the central nervous system, certain microbes have been suggested to cause MS by making a dangerous imprint on the immune system. One way they could do this is by presenting the immune system with substances that look very similar to something in myelin. In such a case, a specific immune reaction against the microbe might inadvertently also attack the body's own myelin. Again, however, there is no evidence that anything like this happens in people with MS. After all, if a bacterium or virus would have caused a 'dangerous' immune reaction which could attack myelin as well, and which would cause MS, the presence of this immune reaction should distinguish people with MS from those without the condition. As pointed out before in this chapter, there is no such difference. As far as we know, there is no virus or bacterium that can be considered as the direct cause of MS.

Chronic cerebrospinal venous insufficiency—CCSVI

Recently, much attention has been drawn to the idea that restricted flow of blood away from the brain would cause MS. This problem, termed 'chronic cerebrospinal venous insufficiency' (CCSVI), is suggested to be the result of certain veins in the neck not being formed properly at birth. When such partially blocked veins would hamper proper drainage of the brain, waste products could conceivably accumulate and cause problems, including MS. The evidence that such blocked veins are only found in people with MS, however, is weak. There is also little evidence for restricted blood flow in that part of the body as such, for whatever reason.

The initial study on CCSVI from Italy suggested that all people with MS had the typical malformations of CCSVI, while none of the control people without MS did. Such a 100% black-and-white difference would be rather remarkable. However, essentially every other study on the subject that has been done since, has revealed a much weaker link. It is now clear that quite a few people with MS do not show any signs of CCSVI, and that many people without MS do. It is therefore certainly not the one and only cause of MS as originally claimed, if it is involved at all.

In the follow-up of the initial claims that CCSVI would cause MS, an intervention was designed to alleviate the blockade in neck veins. This invasive procedure was termed 'liberation treatment'. To date, however, most neurologists would advise against this procedure, unless when it is performed as part of a properly controlled clinical trial. The treatment is certainly not without risks, and its effectiveness in ameliorating any of the symptoms of MS has yet to be demonstrated. To date, the weight of the evidence seems to argue against CCSVI as a cause of MS. Awaiting further developments, let's go back to some older ideas, and examine to what extent they can help us identify the cause of MS.

Are toxic substances to blame?

Just as an infection of myelin-forming cells could stress them, make them accumulate protective substances, and provoke an immune attack, physical trauma such as head injuries or toxic substances could do this too. Regarding physical trauma such as concussions or more serious physical brain damage, we can be brief. There is no indication that this may cause MS. People falling off their bikes or down the stairs do not develop MS more often than anyone else. It has been examined and there is no link between the two.

With regard to toxic chemicals, there is certainly no shortage of ideas for candidates. Toxic barium, rape seed oil, wood-preserving chemicals, toxic moulds, methanol, anything that might be toxic to our brains immediately qualifies. This is a quite a wide range of substances. Many of such toxic substances tend to be around more often, and at higher levels, in industrialized Western societies as compared to tropical areas. Indeed, in the areas where MS is most prevalent. To date, it is difficult to categorically rule out any of them since in almost all cases, we do not have sufficient data to draw any firm final conclusion. In these debates, one candidate toxic substance keeps coming back, and this is dental amalgam.

The claims that dental amalgam may cause MS are based on circumstantial or anecdotal evidence. The idea, for example, that MS appeared to emerge as a distinct disease in the mid 1800s, precisely at the time when dentists started to use amalgam as a filling substance. Another imaginative argument was that Japanese people would have much less MS due to their habit of drinking lots of caries-preventing green tea. No fillings for them, therefore, and no MS either. Or that the prevalence of MS matches the distribution of dentists, as first noted in Hungary. Although the distribution of MS probably also matches that of cinemas and cash machines, this in itself is no reason to immediately discard all observed associations in this context.

Dental amalgam

Dental amalgam is made up of several metals including silver, tin, copper, and zinc. Notably, it also contains substantial amounts of mercury, a toxic metal.

The slightly older reader may remember mercury from the events that took place in the 1950s in the Japanese town of Minamata. Due to the release of mercury-containing waste water from a local plant, mercury poisoning occurred on a massive scale. It ultimately affected almost 3000 people, and killed hundreds. These dramatic events made it abundantly clear that mercury is really quite toxic. In addition, exposure to mercury has been linked to other neurological diseases, pointing to the possibility that the central nervous system may be particularly sensitive to it. Mercury spoiling in Minamata, however, has never been linked to any subsequent increase of MS in the area. MS is rather uncommon in Japan and any mercury-triggered outbreak of MS in Minamata following the disaster should certainly have attracted attention. It has not.

This already casts doubt on the idea that mercury poisoning could cause MS. If it could, one would certainly have expected many more Japanese people around the town of Minamata to have developed the condition. Research data additionally cast doubt on a causative effect of mercury. Admittedly, such studies are not simple to perform. One problem is obviously that not everyone has had fillings of the same composition, the same number of them, or for the same length of time. While studying the effects of dental fillings, people that have them are usually treated as a single group, or at best divided into having few, or many fillings. None of the studies actually measure levels of mercury being released from these filling into the bloodstream, so they are problematic from the start. While keeping this in mind, all literature reports have so far revealed only a very weak link between amalgam fillings and MS. The link is so weak, that by generally accepted standards it does not qualify as being 'statistically significant'. Let's briefly explain what this means. Especially in the study of human health, we are confronted with many factors that may or may not have an effect on a particular health issue. In order to avoid continuous battles between those who claim that a certain effect is meaningful, and others who claim not, the term 'statistical significance' was introduced. It is an agreement that we call something 'statistically significant' if the numbers that come out on any relationship or difference is beyond what may be expected for a chance event. At the same time, a chance event is defined as having a probability of more than 5%. Anything less likely than that is considered unusual and, therefore, potentially meaningful. This is what we call 'statistically significant'. Even something that can be statistically significant may not necessarily be very relevant. When the state of health of large numbers of people is examined for a possible link with lots of different factors, we may easily find very small, meaningless effects to still be 'statistically significant'.

Taking these rules, the available studies on dental fillings consistently fail to reveal an association with MS beyond what may be just a chance event. As far as we know today, dental amalgam does not cause MS.

Can food cause MS?

Sufficient data support the notion that certain parts of our diet may reduce the MS risk, as explained later on. The question whether any type of food may actually cause the condition, is quite another. Some years ago, the idea emerged that a protein in milk could trigger an immune reaction that could cross-react with myelin. It led some to think that consuming milk or other dairy products could mislead the immune system into an attack on myelin, and thus contribute to MS. We don't think so. Drinking milk does not immediately provoke an immune reaction against milk proteins. Drinking milk is much more likely to make you tolerant for any protein in milk. It activates the system of peripheral tolerance. There is no evidence that any immune reaction contributes to MS. Especially when it has been fortified with vitamin D, drinking milk is not something one should avoid to prevent or cure MS.

Also other food components such as gluten, legumes (beans, soy, peanuts, peas, etc.), and anything with high levels of sugar have been declared dangerous. Again, however, the evidence that these products cause MS or make it worse, is unconvincing. The same applies to hormones or antibiotics in our food.

More recently, studies have started to focus on the bacteria that live in our gut. Dairy products and fermented food supply us with enormous numbers of harmless bacteria that persist in our gut. By looking more closely at these bacteria, researchers are currently trying to examine in what way they may influence our immune system. It is quite possible that specific types of gut bacteria may predispose to chronic inflammation, while others may perhaps protect against it. To date, however, much has still to be learned on this subject.

Further reading

Aminzadeh KK and Etminan M (2007) Dental amalgam and multiple sclerosis: a systematic review and meta-analysis. *J Public Health Dent* **67**: 64–6.

McFarland HF and Martin R (2008) Multiple sclerosis: a complicated picture of autoimmunity. *Nat Immunol* **8**: 913–19.

Steinman L (2009) A molecular trio in relapse and remission in multiple sclerosis. *Nat Rev Immunol* **9**: 440–7.

Van der Valk P and Amor S (2009) Preactive lesions in multiple sclerosis. *Curr Opin Neurol* **22**: 207–13.

7

Which drugs may help suppress MS?

→ Key Points

◆ Several MS drugs can slow down the activity and progression of MS. In the next few years, more drugs with such effects will become available, including new oral drugs. Most of them influence the immune system, some impact on brain functions.

◆ While offering some relief, current MS drugs may also cause side effects. They suppress immune functions in a general way, and this may lead to a reduced ability of the immune system to fight off infections and tumours in the long run, or perform its reparative role. The search for more selective drugs continues.

For a long time, people with MS have been faced with the reality that no effective treatment for their condition was available. This has changed, and several drugs are now available to slow down MS. The development of novel and more specific drugs will continue, since current drugs rather indiscriminately tone down the immune system as a whole. While this may well slow down the activity and progression of MS, the long-term effects of blocking or inhibiting immune functions are of concern. After all, the useful side of the immune system is also suppressed by these drugs. Further improvements may therefore come from drugs that specifically target the cause of MS, or the parts of the immune system that really matter, while allowing other parts to continue with their job of defending us against infections and tumours. In this chapter, we will discuss the MS drugs that are approved, and explain how these drugs are thought to work. There are also several new drugs in development, not yet approved, that are worth mentioning. We will not comment too much about current drug benefits. Not only may these benefits be variable from one person with MS to the next, the more recent MS drugs especially have been used for too short a period of time to make final statements, particularly on their long-term benefits and side effects.

In the context of discussing drugs for MS, we also briefly explain what it takes to develop a new drug. When newspapers report about exciting research that identifies a potential new drug for MS, it is usually mentioned that it will take at least another 'five years or so' before it could be on the market. Why is that? What stops people from making such exciting new drugs available straight away? We will explain why this is, and what happens during the 'five years or so'.

Apart from traditional drugs that come from pharmaceutical and biotech laboratories, a highly creative range of other alternative or complementary interventions continue to be tried. Especially at the time that no conventional drugs were available to help people with MS, many other potential cures were designed and tested. These include special diets, homeopathy, herbal medicine, acupuncture, osteopathy, chiropractic, aromatherapy, bee venom treatment, goat serum, experimental stem cell therapies, and other non-conventional approaches. We will discuss these in the next chapter.

Why does it take another 'five years or so'?

One reason that the development of conventional drugs takes such a long time are the bad experiences we had in the past, when new drugs were allowed to reach patients much more quickly than today. In the 1960s, for example, the now infamous drug thalidomide, widely used in Europe for morning sickness in pregnant women, unexpectedly caused serious birth defects. Over 10,000 children were born with missing or deformed limbs due to their mothers having used thalidomide during pregnancy. That drugs could have such effects created a big shock. As a result, strict rules were designed to ensure this would never happen again. From then on, all new drugs had to be much more rigorously tested before being allowed onto the market. Yet, nasty side effects of new experimental drugs continue to surprise us, prompting authorities to continuously design even stricter rules. The agencies that make sure that these rules are obeyed include the European Medicines Agency (EMA), and the Food and Drug Administration (FDA) in the US. Without their approval, drugs are simply not allowed onto the market.

The current rules are very strict indeed. Before allowing any new drug on the market, its manufacturing process is scrutinized in great detail, and the drug will have to be first tested on laboratory animals. Quantities of the drug administered in these tests are much larger than will be intended for patients. There are very strict rules on how such tests are to be conducted, and how the paperwork that documents the results needs to be drawn up. If anything bad happens at this stage, the development of the drug stops immediately. When the animal tests are OK, the drug is then tested on healthy volunteers using quantities far below those already known to be safe for animals. This is called a Phase I test. It is not meant to test whether the drug does anything useful, but only to see if it harms humans.

If the Phase I test is good, the new drug is then tested in a small group of patients it is designed for, since patients may respond differently to a drug from healthy people. Such a first patient test is called a Phase II test, and primarily aims to confirm its safety also in patients, of the benefits hoped for, and to establish a drug dose that achieves useful effects. Finally, a Phase III test is required to test the new drug at an active dose in a much larger group of patients. Usually, this involves hundreds of people in different countries. This final test must confirm that it actually works, and to what extent.

The importance of also testing a fake drug, a placebo

In both Phase II and Phase III tests, the effect of the new drug on patients is usually compared to a fake drug, also called placebo. In MS trials, an existing drug can be taken for comparison too. A new drug has to show benefit over placebo, and preferably also over existing drugs. Comparing the different treatments is done in a way that neither the patient nor the doctor knows whether they are working with the real drug, or with the placebo or comparator drug. This way of doing things is called 'double-blind'. It is to prevent either patient or doctor being influenced by a certain expectation or hope when performing EDSS or MSIS-29 scoring, or when examining MRI scans to evaluate the clinical effects. Frequently, people with chronic diseases will feel better because of the beneficial effects of the extra care and attention they receive during a trial. The doctors may sympathize with their patients to the extent that they too become influenced by their hopes or expectations when evaluating results. This is called 'the placebo effect', and it is not something to ignore. In fact, tests in MS have shown it to be real, despite that you might think it is only self-delusional. It is not. For several people with MS, simply taking part in a Phase II or III test even when they are given only placebo, already makes them do better. Yet, it obviously does not mean that the drug treatment as such was of any use, since in a placebo group, there actually is none.

Only after a successful Phase III test, using a double-blinded set-up, will EMA or FDA allow new drugs onto the market. The complete procedure takes many years and vast sums of money. Especially in MS, it is impossible to establish the effects of new drugs or treatment overnight. MS symptoms only gradually increase, or indeed, spontaneously decrease sometimes without doing anything. In addition, the effects of certain drugs may take some time to kick in. For these reasons, it may take many years before we can be sure that a new MS drug really works. While the rules are therefore very strict, they are there to ensure that no drugs are made available that could actually harm people, or do not have any objective effect at all.

Importantly, the rules and requirements are not just there to protect patients from potentially dangerous drugs. They also reflect the generally accepted set of requirements for calling any drug or therapy effective. The term 'evidence-based medicine' is commonly used to refer to these requirements. Essentially, it means that professionals in the field agree that for any drug to be considered useful and worthy of financial compensation, there must be reliable and objective evidence for a sufficient beneficial effect, to be acquired by research complying with the previously described rules. In the absence of such evidence, one could go on arguing about possible benefits forever. Respecting the standards of proper clinical research is particularly important in MS, with its variable symptoms that often spontaneously change over short periods of time. Especially then, long-term testing on large groups of people, taking the 'placebo effect' into account, is the only way to establish whether something works or not. In the absence of this discipline, honest enthusiasm or commercial interests could easily take over.

Which conventional drugs exist to treat MS?

Drugs that are currently approved for use in MS include variants of interferon-beta, glatiramer acetate, mitoxantrone, natalizumab, and fingolimod. In the following sections we briefly describe these drugs, and explain how they are thought to work. Procedures for acquiring FDA and EMA approval for several other drugs are ongoing. It is reasonable to expect that the number of approved MS drugs will grow in the next few years. Apart from these dedicated MS drugs, serious relapses in MS are still treated with steroids, general anti-inflammatory drugs which help reduce inflammation. These substances, including (methyl)prednisolone or cortisone, are very powerful drugs which suppress immune cells. They are only meant as a short-term treatment, to reduce the intensity of a relapse and to speed recovery. They do not change the outcome of a relapse, nor the long-term course of MS. Because steroids are so powerful, they also have quite a few side effects. For this reason, steroids are generally not used for longer than 3 weeks, and for no more than three times a year.

Interferon-beta

In 1987, the results were published of a small trial in which people with MS were treated with interferon-gamma, a natural substance produced by immune cells, which helps the immune system fight infections. At that time, many believed that MS was caused by a viral infection, even despite the fact that no 'MS virus' had been identified. Boosting the immune system's activity to kill viruses was therefore expected to suppress the disease, no matter what the virus might be. In fact, the reverse was found. People given interferon-gamma rapidly experienced worsening of their MS symptoms. This failed test was immediately stopped, but it led researchers to examine the effects of another interferon, known to have effects opposite to those of interferon-gamma. A few years later, this substance, called interferon-beta, was indeed found to have some beneficial effects, albeit not in all people with MS. Interferon-beta is produced in two different variations, called 1a and 1b. These variants are supplied under trade names currently including Avonex®, Rebif®, Cinnovex™, Betaseron®, Ziferon™, and Extavia®.

Like the natural form of interferon-beta produced by our bodies, the drug version has a wide range of effects on the immune system. One prominent effect appears to be that blood vessels in the brain and spinal cord are 'fortified' making it more difficult for immune cells to enter the central nervous system. Also, interferon-beta makes T cells changes their colour code to yellow. This code is explained in the chapter on the immune system. The substances that 'code yellow' T cells produce tone down immune reactions, instead of stimulating them. More properties of interferon-beta include the ability to induce endorphins, slow down the activity of tissue-degrading enzymes, reduce amounts of MHC proteins on macrophages, and to make activated T cells die more quickly. It is probably because of this wide variety of mild effects acting together, that people with MS respond differently to the drug.

Glatiramer acetate

Glatiramer acetate, also known as Copaxone®, is quite an unusual drug. Rather than a single substance, like most drugs are, it is a collection of artificial proteins. The idea of using it for MS originated in Israel, as the result of studies using the mouse model of MS. In mice, MS-like symptoms can be induced by injections of brain-derived materials. In an attempt to replace brain-derived materials with a more simple synthetic substance, glatiramer acetate was tried. It is not really a single substance, but a mixture of substances. It was supposed to mimic one of the most abundant proteins in the myelin sheath. Surprisingly, however, it did not induce the MS-like disease in mice, as expected, but stopped it from developing instead. Without knowing exactly why this effect occurred, it was then decided to test glatiramer acetate in people with MS.

The way glatiramer acetate works is still largely unknown. The overall composition of the artificial proteins roughly resembles that of a protein that is found in myelin, but only roughly. While this has led to suggestions that it could act as a decoy for the autoimmune attack, there is no clear evidence to support his idea. The cells of the immune system that matter most in this context tend to be very specific. It seems unlikely that they would confuse glatiramer acetate with actual proteins in myelin. Instead, there are some indications that glatiramer acetate may change the previously mentioned colour codes, or other features of T cells.

Mitoxantrone

Also known as Novantrone®, mitoxantrone, an anti-cancer drug, has also been used to slow down MS. As can be expected from an anti-cancer drug, mitoxantrone prevents cells from multiplying. It does so in tumour cells, but also other cells, including adaptive immune cells. Under normal conditions, an immune response relies on multiplication of those cells to fight off the emerging danger. By preventing them from doing so, immune responses, including autoimmune responses, are therefore dampened. This is the way mitoxantrone helps to dampen MS attacks.

Unfortunately, stopping cells from multiplying altogether is very unhealthy in the long run. Our body needs cells to multiply all the time to keep up with the necessary repairs and replacements, and to make our immune system function properly. Treatment with mitoxantrone can therefore be continued for only 2–3 years, and with a limited total number of doses. Once someone has received a certain total amount of the drug, it can no longer be given, not even after a long time. It would otherwise cause too much damage to the body. Clearly, it is not a long-term solution.

Natalizumab

Natalizumab, also called Tysabri®, is an artificially made antibody, and like other antibodies, it can stick to something tightly. Natalizumab is designed to selectively stick to the surface of immune cells so they can no longer leave the blood circulation to go into tissues. As explained before, and illustrated in Fig. 7.1, immune cells attach to blood vessel walls by using a Velcro-like system. 'Hooks' on the surface of immune cells catch 'loops' on blood vessel walls. Only when immune cells are properly caught by the vessel wall, can they start squeezing their way out of the vessel, into the brain for example.

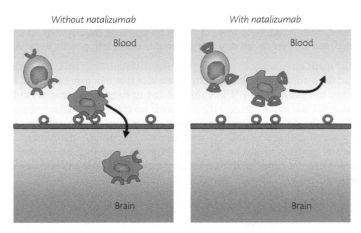

Fig. 7.1 Natalizumab blocks immune cells from going into the brain.

When the 'hooks' on immune cells become covered with a sticky substance such as natalizumab, they cannot attach to the 'loops' anymore, and are blocked from entering the brain or spinal cord. As a result, the immune cells can no longer become recruited by the brain or spinal cord, and drive the local immune reactions that cause the damage in MS. Using this strategy, natalizumab is used to slow down the destructive process in MS.

Fingolimod

Fingolimod, also referred to as FTY720, is the most recently approved drug for MS and the first oral drug. It is marketed under the trade name Gilenya®. It is now an option for those who do not respond very well to treatment with either interferon or glatiramer acetate. Once taken up by the body, fingolimod's structure changes slightly. The new chemical substance formed binds to a certain type of receptor on cells. This blocks the function of the receptor, and makes it disappear from the cell surface. Among the many types of cells that carry fingolimod's target receptor are immune cells. When fingolimod interferes with the receptor on immune cells, these cells are hampered in their normal movement from lymph nodes and spleen into the bloodstream. As a result, immune cells get stuck in those organs, and become much less likely to reach the brain or spinal cord. This clearly lowers the chance that they might contribute to the inflammatory damage in MS.

The effect of fingolimod on immune cells is only part of the story. The receptor it affects is found on many cells, not just immune cells, and its function on these different cells is not always the same. Many cells in the brain and spinal cord also carry fingolimod's target receptor. Nerve cells, for example, do, and astrocytes, important support cells in the central nervous system. Since fingolimod is also able to enter the central nervous system, these other cells may be affected as well. This does not necessarily mean that this is a problem. In fact, recent studies in animals indicate that fingolimod's effects on astrocytes may contribute to its beneficial effects on MS. Yet, many cell types may be affected by fingolimod, and most of fingolimod's effects are still not fully known. Its use will therefore continue to require careful monitoring for a long time still.

Side effects

Most of the side effects of interferon and glatiramer acetate are well known, as these drugs have now been used for many years. Both drugs can cause injection site reactions, like pain and some swelling. Interferon can induce some flu-like symptoms, while glatiramer acetate can lead to disappearance of body fat under the skin at the injection site. Apart from this latter effect which is permanent, most of these side effects resolve spontaneously, and do not cause any long-term issues. The situation is somewhat different for the newer drugs. Natalizumab

(Tysabri®) and fingolimod (FTY720) are markedly more effective than the older drugs in slowing down MS, at least in the short term. Yet, there is a potentially dark side to their effects, which should also be acknowledged.

Both natalizumab and fingolimod stop immune cells going into the brain and spinal cord, although they achieve this in different ways. It must be remembered, however, that immune cells continuously leave blood vessels and enter tissues and organs including the brain and spinal cord, for a very good reason. They need to clear infections and tumours, and also need to stop ongoing immune responses, as well as promote repair of any damage. If immune cells are continuously blocked from doing so by a drug, infections or tumours may not be sufficiently kept in check any longer, and repair of damage might also become compromised. After all, these drugs work indiscriminately in their actions. They target all immune cells, irrespective of their function. That this might cause unintended trouble was emphasized after natalizumab appeared on the market. A few people that used both natalizumab in combination with other drugs developed a very aggressive and deadly infection in the brain. The virus which caused this is a normal resident in many people's brains, but natalizumab can block the immune system from keeping it in check. Present data indicate that this happens in approximately one in every 600 people. Only after careful review of all the data by the FDA was natalizumab allowed back onto the market but only under certain conditions, which were stricter than before. It is not to be used with other MS drugs, and only as a last resort. Concerns over its long-term effects remain.

Information on possible side effects of fingolimod is still limited to the short-term effects that were observed during the recent clinical trials. Even over this limited period of time, some clues emerged that immune control over viruses, in this case herpes viruses, may be reduced. While much remains to be established, the relatively strong effects of natalizumab and fingolimod on the course of MS emphasize the need to monitor not only the beneficial effects of such drugs, but also their potential side effects in the long run.

Which other drug treatments are emerging?

There is a wide array of new candidate drugs that continue to be developed and tested for MS. We will mention only a few here, since there are too many to describe in detail. Please visit the websites of the National MS Societies of the USA or UK which provide lists of ongoing trials, and a brief description of the ideas behind them (see the reference to useful websites at the end of this book). You will find that even existing drugs are continuously being re-tested in new modes of administration, in adjusted quantities, or in combination with other drugs.

Among new drugs that are at advanced stages of testing are several antibody-based drugs which, like natalizumab, stick to immune cells to block a particular activity. Some of these not only stick to their target cell, but actually kill it too. One of these drugs, called rituximab, targets and kills B cells. This has beneficial effects in MS, at least in the short term. B cells are immune cells that ultimately develop into antibody-producing cells, but they fulfil other roles as well. Rituximab does not change the levels of antibodies very much. Its effect on MS therefore most likely results from eliminating the antigen-presenting function of B cells. Interfering with B cells, however, does not always produce the same effect. The use of aticacept, another drug that targets B-cells, led to increased inflammatory activity in people with MS. Trials with this product were therefore halted.

Another therapeutic antibody in development is alemtuzumab (Lemtrada^{TM}, also known as Campath$^®$). This antibody sticks to immune cells, including T cells, and kills them. It was tested in MS already many years ago, and continues to be tested, especially as an early treatment and for people who do not respond to interferon. Yet more specific antibodies are being developed and tested, most of them based on the same principle of attaching to immune cells and either killing them, or blocking key functions of such cells. Daclizumab is another example; it attaches to the surface of T cells and prevents them from multiplying.

Apart from specific antibody-based therapies, several other general immune-modulatory drugs such as teriflunomide and fumarate are currently under investigation. These are all artificial small molecules which have the major advantage of being oral drugs. They are in the final stages of testing, and results so far generally appear to be encouraging. While some of their biological effects are known, the full range of the impact of these drugs on the body, and the extent of their side effects, is yet to be established. At least some of these new products are expected to reach the market in the near future, research into these products will continue, to find out more on exactly how they work. The path towards new MS drugs, however, is full of pitfalls. In 2011, the experimental drugs cladribine and laquinimod both failed to reach the standards set at the very last stage of their clinical testing. This only emphasizes the surprises that still remain around the corner, and underpins the need for close scrutiny of all new MS drugs for a long time to come still.

Low-dose naltrexone

Naltrexone is a good example of how the high costs of drug development can work against a potentially useful substance in the absence of patent protection. As explained, it takes vast sums of money to develop and test a drug, especially in a condition which requires long-term monitoring such as MS. It is understandable that few are willing to cover the costs of testing a compound which is no longer commercially protected. Here's naltrexone. It is for sale at a price that is within a child's pocket money budget.

Naltrexone is a small artificial substance, which resembles the natural opium-like substances that the brain uses itself. It was approved by the FDA some 25 years ago to help heroin addicts. Heroin activates a lock-and-key mechanism in the brain that triggers nerve cells into experiencing the 'pleasures' of the drug. By taking its place in this lock-and-key mechanism but not triggering nerve cells, naltrexone blocks the effects of heroin. It takes away the 'fun' when taken at high doses. At low doses, naltrexone does activate nerve cells for a short while, and gives a little bit of the 'heroin effect'. In response to low-dose naltrexone, nerve cells produce endorphins, morphine-like substances that act to dampen the effects of pain and provide a feeling of general well-being. People generally like having endorphins in their brain. Apart from acting as a pain killer, they also slow down the activity of the immune system. Many people with MS have reported improvement in the quality of their life as the result of these effects.

No large-scale trials have yet been conducted to objectively confirm the several anecdotal reports on the favourable effects of low-dose naltrexone. A recent small-scale trial in Italy has focused on primary-progressive MS. The results of this trial indicate that a daily low dose of naltrexone is safe, and strengthens the build-up of endorphins in the blood of people with MS. The trial was not designed to monitor long-term effects of MS, leaving the final verdict on low-dose naltrexone to the future.

Cannabis

Finally, cannabinoids, the active ingredients of cannabis, are worth mentioning. They are in the same league as low-dose naltrexone since they also influence natural signalling systems in the brain. Like low-dose naltrexone, cannabinoids have proven beneficial effects on muscle spasms and pain, major symptoms of MS for some people. For this reason, they should not be considered as non-conventional drugs as, for example, acupuncture, homeopathy, or bee venom therapy. For the latter, there is no objective evidence that they are effective. For cannabis, this is much clearer. Yet, the use of cannabis is obviously 'non-conventional' in that it does have some clear negative side effects, and is politically controversial. Also, it is difficult to obtain cannabis of a constant quality. The cultivar that is used, the way it is grown, and even the time of day it is harvested can markedly influence its precise composition, and levels of the active substance tetrahydrocannabinol, or THC. Yet, much is already known about the way cannabinoids ease spasms and pain. The brain actually uses very similar substances itself to achieve the same effect. Given its undeniable effects, therefore, research continues into the design of cannabis-like substances that can be produced with a constant quality, and applied with the same beneficial effects, but without the intrinsic variability, side effects, or indeed, political ramifications.

Concluding remarks

The list of emerging new treatments and drugs for MS illustrates that we are not there yet when it comes to treating MS. Many variant drugs are emerging which tone down the immune system, each in their own way. The ultimate challenge remains to unravel the process that causes MS, and to clarify which substance in the brain and spinal cord provokes the damaging immune response. When this substance is found, a treatment may be designed which switches off the immune response to this particular substance, without interfering with the rest of the immune system. It would be like wielding a scalpel rather than a hammer. There are ways to do this, by using the principles of immune tolerance, explained in the chapter on the immune system. Consider such an approach as 'reverse vaccination'. It is not aimed at building up an immune response against a defined target, like a vaccine does, but instead, at the elimination of one. Such approaches could perhaps help avoid the side effects of current drugs that influence the entire immune system. Research towards this goal continues.

Further reading

Baker D, Jackson SJ, and Pryce G (2007) Cannabinoid control of neuroinflammation related to multiple sclerosis. *Br J Pharmacol* 15: 649–54.

Compston A and Coles A (2008) Multiple sclerosis. *Lancet* 372: 1502–17.

Lutterotti A and Martin R (2008) Getting specific: monoclonal antibodies in multiple sclerosis. *Lancet Neurol* 7: 537–47.

Kieseier BC, Wiendl H, Leussink VI, *et al* (2008) Immunomodulatory treatment strategies in multiple sclerosis. *J Neurol* 255 (S6): 15–21.

Gironi M, Martinelli-Boneschi F, Sacerdote P, *et al* (2008) A pilot trial of low-dose naltrexone in primary progressive multiple sclerosis. *Mult Scler* 14: 1076–83.

8

Which non-conventional treatments may help suppress MS?

> **Key Points**
>
> - Most alternative or complementary forms of medicine have never been properly tested in MS by double-blind, placebo-controlled clinical studies. We therefore have no data to show that they work.
>
> - Stem cells hold significant promise for therapy, but routine stem cell treatment of MS is not possible yet.
>
> - The possible benefits or risks of surgical intervention in chronic cerebrospinal venous insufficiency are not fully clarified yet, and require further studies.
>
> - With only one exception, nothing other than general rules for a healthy diet apply to someone with MS, as they do to everyone else.
>
> - The exception is vitamin D, which has marked beneficial effects on MS irrespective of drug use. It not only reduces the risk of developing MS in the first place, but makes relapses occur less frequently once MS has started. Everyone with MS should consider taking extra vitamin D, especially in winter.

It is an attractive idea to suppress MS symptoms by changing lifestyles, diets, or fairly innocent interventions like aromatherapy, homeopathy, or acupuncture. Even certain treatments advertised as 'stem cell transplantations', or 'liberation treatments' may be better than doing nothing. At this point, we return to the point of 'evidence-based medicine' made in the previous chapter, since the debate on non-conventional ways to treat MS is often confused by misunderstandings. Researchers and clinicians in one camp, and alternative healers in another, seem to speak different languages. More often than not, different standards are used to judge the validity of information or claims.

Without agreement over the way one should judge whether a treatment or lifestyle change has any merit in helping people with MS, any debate on a given treatment will likely remain unproductive. It is therefore useful to clarify how researchers and clinicians judge information, and why they do this in a particular way.

When considering the possible effectiveness of a treatment on MS, researchers and clinicians adhere to certain rules. They are trained to understand how useful information should be obtained, and when valid conclusions can be drawn. Importantly, they also learn when one cannot draw any conclusions from an experiment or data sets. They use words like 'theories', 'hypotheses', 'controls', 'statistical significance', to describe the rules they respect. These rules do not reflect any personal preference, but they are of universal validity. All researchers use the same rules, all over the world, and they have been doing so for centuries, ever since the ancient Greeks started formulating these rules, which they called 'logic'. They guide us in acquiring new and valid knowledge about the world around us. Just like mathematics leaves no space for personal preferences, the rules of logic are also non-negotiable.

People involved with non-conventional or complementary therapies in MS often seem to have difficulties in respecting the rules of logic. An important rule of logic for example is: 'When trying to prove your idea wrong or right, you must always leave space to find out that your idea might be wrong'. Don't just focus on being right, therefore, even if you are convinced that you are. This is why proper experiments must always include a 'negative control', or in the case of clinical studies, a placebo, a fake drug. If you do not allow space to find out that the result of your intervention would have been the same without any intervention at all, the results are obviously meaningless. It is like performing a rain dance. The rain will inevitably come someday, but you might as well have spent your time reading a decent book instead of dancing. This point is particularly important in the case of MS, with its relapses and remissions. In general, it is more likely for someone to seek an alternative cure or treatment when things are at their worst, during a relapse therefore. Consequently, it is likely that even by doing nothing useful at all, improvement follows because relapses tend to fade anyway. Spontaneous remissions in MS may thus easily be confused with the effect of a mysterious cure.

When reviewing data on the various strategies used in alternative or complementary medicine, the conclusion is that there is not enough proper data to suggest that any of them are helpful in MS. To be fair, it is understandable that non-conventional interventions are usually not tested in clinical trials. Such trials are very expensive, and in the absence of any commercial protection of the final product or treatment, who is going to pay for that? Also, design of a placebo group is frequently problematic in the case of alternative treatments. It is difficult to fake acupuncture, and a traditional homeopathic treatment is already a placebo itself. However, these considerations still do not justify ignoring the rules of logic. Aromatherapy, chiropractic, acupuncture, homeopathy, bee-venom therapy, and similar treatments may be relatively harmless, but there is no good evidence to think that they may improve the condition of people with MS.

Stem cell treatment

Over recent years, mainstream research has become intrigued by the prospect of using stem cell technology to cure diseases. Mind-boggling images of a mouse with a newly grown ear on its back have captured the imagination of many.

Originally, some believed that stem cells would be used for reconstruction of entire tissues and organs in a culture dish, so they could be transplanted into patients to replace any damaged organ. Indeed, laboratory experiments have shown striking examples of how cells in a culture dish can grow into throbbing heart tissue, or into a layer of skin. Would it not be great to do this with brain or spinal cord tissue? While individual human brain cells can indeed be kept in a culture dish, as shown in Fig. 8.1, growing an entire brain is quite

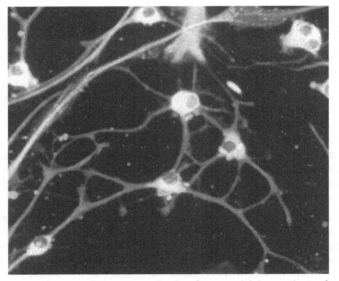

Fig. 8.1 Not only stem cells, but even cells taken from an adult human brain after death can be made to multiply in the laboratory. However, using them for therapy is an entirely different matter.

a different story. The ear on the mouse, by the way was just new skin growing over a plastic mould which made it look like an ear. To get rid of some more nonsense: growing a new brain or spinal cord to replace a damaged one is obviously ludicrous.

The next best idea is to replace the small parts of the brain and spinal cord that are damaged in MS. The problem, however, is that these parts are scattered all over the brain and spinal cord. Each of the damaged sites needs to be dealt with individually. Also, most of the damaged spots have turned into scar tissue, which would refuse to make way for any newly growing tissue. And how would one reconnect the long nerve fibres that once ran there? For these reasons, chances to replace any of the sites of existing MS scars with functional new tissue are minimal.

When considering the options in MS, the real hope seems to be that stem cells may be used to limit damage in progress, and to promote the formation of new myelin. Stem cells grow enthusiastically, but they also act as little factories for many substances that promote growth and repair. Also, they can regulate immune responses. Rather than trying to grow new functional brain or spinal cord tissue from stem cells, these cells are probably more useful as local 'drug factories'. They release natural substances to tone down immune reactions and assist the healing process. This more general immune-modulatory effect of certain types of stem cells will probably turn out to be the easiest to explore. Indeed, clinical trials to test stem cells in this application are currently being conducted.

Replacing damaged tissue remains a different issue. Experiments in animals show that some stem cells can help promote the formation of new myelin at sites of progressing damage. Other experiments show that stem cells may even find their way to sites of active damage when administered into the bloodstream. These encouraging findings raise the hope that one day, stem cells may indeed also be used to help control damage in scattered and largely inaccessible places such as the brain and spinal cord, for as long as the damage is ongoing. The road to application of these strategies is still long, and probably full of pitfalls. We do not know what the behaviour of these stem cells will be when they enter the scene of an active immune reaction, as in MS. This is of particular concern since we do not really know yet which factors drive the immune reaction in MS to begin with. Remember that in people with MS, the brain very often does attempt to repair the damage done by immune reactions. Yet, this repair process somehow fails. How will stem cells respond, if the natural mechanisms to make new myelin have already failed? Why would stem cells succeed? How will they respond to the apparently hostile environment they will encounter? Will they become immediately targeted themselves, and only provide more fuel for the fire? Will they be stimulated in such a way that they will grow into tumours, rather than into useful myelin-forming cells?

How long are they going to survive for? These are issues that will have to be worked out before stems cells can be routinely applied in the clinic. It will still take some years before we get to the point that safe stem cell therapies can be routinely implemented. Several trials are ongoing, but private clinics that offer 'stem cell treatment' for significant amounts of money are best ignored.

In summary, the perspective that stem cell therapy may one day be useful in MS is realistic. Impressive advances in animal models have shown the ability of stem cells to control immune reactions, and promote repair of damaged myelin. At the same time, the way stem cells will behave in the context of MS is still largely the subject of speculation. Various types of stem cells exist, each with their own theoretical advantages and disadvantages. Human adults are no laboratory rats. We are not there yet. Until we understand more of the behaviour of stem cells, and what to expect when we inject them into people with MS, being patient appears to be the most sensible thing to do.

Can certain diets suppress MS?

There are few subjects more difficult to examine than the effect of food on health, or indeed, on chronic diseases. One reason is that food is so complex in composition, that it is almost impossible to define precisely what is in it. In addition, we know that the biological effects of certain substances in our food are influenced by other substances in food. Certain vitamins, for example, are taken up by the body more rapidly, or more slowly, in the presence of certain food components. Also, our body adapts to food. When you eat something every day, your body grows used to it, and builds up specific enzymes to quickly deal with it next time. Switching between certain types of food therefore produces different effects from eating something every day. Quantities of food make a difference too, since the effects of certain components depend very much on quantity. Think of vitamins. They are generally essential for good health, but may actually cause toxic effects if you exaggerate their consumption. Finally, we have enormous numbers of different bacteria in the gut, literally billions. These bacteria influence the way the body deals with food, for example, by helping to break down vegetables. If the types of bacteria in your gut change after infection or an antibiotic course, the digestive process will work out differently too. In short, it is a daunting task to make sure what any given type of food or food component actually does, at what dose, in combination with which other type of food, ingested in which frequency, and in which person, at what age. You see the problem.

In Chapter 2, we have already pointed out that certain dietary measures are useful to alleviate bladder or bowel dysfunction in MS. Avoiding caffeine or alcohol, eating regularly and healthily, and ingesting sufficient amounts of fibres are helpful in this context. Yet, in this chapter we address the question whether certain food components can actually prevent MS, or cure it. Given the earlier introduction to this issue, it will probably be no surprise that the answer is a disappointing one. Almost none of the claims that certain types of foods prevent or suppress MS are sufficiently supported by reliable data that take all the previously discussed variables and complications into account. There is simply not enough information to know whether MS-specific health claims of certain fibres, low-carbohydrate, anti-oxidants, alfalfa sprouts, wheat germs, lactic acid bacteria, etc. are valid or not. They probably are not. Vitamins B12, A, and E do not seem to play any special role either. Also the widely repeated claim that omega-3 poly-unsaturated fatty acids are helpful still remains unproven. These fatty acids are generally beneficial to anyone's health, but there is no evidence that they are particularly useful to control MS. Also the idea that leaving out certain ingredients from your diet, such as dairy products, gluten, legumes, or sugar is helpful for people with MS remains unsubstantiated.

There is, however, one exception, and that is vitamin D. We have to immediately state that to the best of our knowledge, a proper clinical study of the effects of vitamin D on MS has not been reported yet. A trial in which vitamin D is given as an add-on to people with MS who are already using interferon, is currently being conducted. The circumstantial evidence for a beneficial effect of vitamin D on MS is impressive. Earlier on, we described the environmental factors that influence the risk for MS, including the effects of sunlight. One of the main effects of sunlight is that it makes the body produce vitamin D. An unhealthy lack of sunlight exposure leads to chronically low levels of vitamin D, and this is associated with an increased risk for MS, an effect that start building up before birth. Apart from sunlight, our body has one other major source of vitamin D, and this is food. It is rapidly becoming clear that the effects of vitamin D in food parallel the effects of sunlight. Other data paint the same picture. Vitamin D tones down aggressive immune functions, and people with MS tend to have lower levels of vitamin D than others. This difference is even seen in younger people up to the age of 20 who developed MS later on in life. It is the accumulation of consistent biological, clinical, epidemiological, and even genetic evidence that really strengthens the case for vitamin D.

The effects of food-derived vitamin D

We have explained how difficult it is to establish the health effects of certain food components. Food is devastatingly complex in composition, and many other factors influence the effects of food substances. Vitamin D, however, is a special case. What makes studying vitamin D easier than other food components, is that vitamin D levels can be measured in blood. This makes it possible to objectively compare aspects of health with actual vitamin D levels. Also, vitamin D is found in very few types of food. Only fatty fish like salmon and mackerel, cod liver oil, egg yolk and certain mushrooms contain meaningful quantities of vitamin D. It is therefore easier to trace in people's feeding habits than many other food components. The amounts of vitamin D in our body is largely the result of how much fatty fish we eat, how much time we spend in the sun, and, of course, how often we ingest vitamin D tablets. Vitamin D has attracted attention for some time already, ever since it was found that it blocks an MS-like disease in laboratory animals just as effectively as some drugs do. Laboratory tests on cells grown in dishes confirm that vitamin D influences immune cells in a way that could easily work favourably in MS. In other words: the laboratory data on vitamin D indicate that it could well impact favourably on MS. The question is: does it?

A convincing clue that vitamin D in food reduces the risk for MS has emerged from Norway. While MS tends to increase with the distance from the equator, both on the northern and southern hemisphere, Norway is an exception to this rule. Marked differences exist in sunlight exposure in northern regions of Norway and its southern parts, but the frequency of MS does not change according to global rules. It unexpectedly decreases about 50% as one goes north. Taking various possible explanations into account, diet appears to be the only convincing factor to explain this. In the coastal regions of northern Norway, people eat unusually large amounts of fatty fish.

Especially trout and salmon are local favourites. In addition, people in this region have a strong tradition of consuming large quantities of cod liver oil in winter. Originally, the protective effect on MS of this rather outspoken fish-eating habit in the area was attributed to poly-unsaturated omega-3 fatty acids. More recent studies have clarified that more likely, it is vitamin D in fish which causes the effect. A dose of up to 4000 units of vitamin D per meal, ten to twenty times what is often quoted as the recommended daily intake for adults, is no oddity on northern Norwegian tables. Because of this, vitamin D is now widely believed to be the factor responsible for the fact that fish-loving Norwegians in the north experience MS much less frequently than one would expect on the basis of their genes and the general lack of sunshine in the area.

While such stories are of interest, it is still no proof. After all, and as stated, food is complicated and people in northern Norway may have other habits that may impact on MS too. Another way to examine whether or not food-derived vitamin D impacts on MS is to track what people are eating, before anyone gets MS to begin with. Such studies are not easy. It involves asking many young people to keep a record of exactly how much vitamin D they eat over a period of years, especially from food supplements. Information on these feeding habits should be supported by actual measurements of vitamin D blood levels. Over time, one could then compare the MS frequency in groups with high intake or low intake of vitamin D. One such study has been done. The results are very clear, and they support the Norwegian tale. Young women who have a high intake of vitamin D over a long period of time, have an MS risk which is substantially lower than those who had taken less vitamin D, well beyond the possible effects of chance.

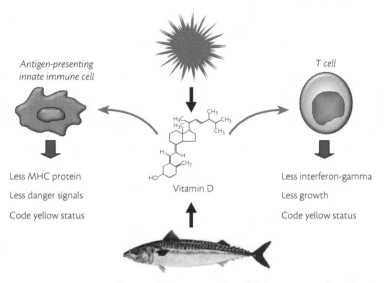

Fig. 8.2 Vitamin D we get from sunlight or eating fatty fish, has a range of beneficial effects including toning down immune responses. Similar to immune-modulating drugs, vitamin D helps to keep MS under control.

These findings on food-derived vitamin D are in perfect agreement with information on the effects of sunlight we discussed before. Sunlight, which also provides the body with vitamin D, also protects from MS, and dampens the disease process. To conclude this chapter, we would therefore like to make a special point about vitamin D. Main sources of vitamin D, and their effects on the immune system, are illustrated in Fig. 8.2.

Please take your vitamin D

It is becoming increasingly clear that vitamin D has a marked protective effect on MS. It reduces the MS risk. More importantly perhaps, recent data suggest that it also reduces the likelihood that someone with MS will experience another relapse. Its effects are like that of an MS drug. So what do we learn from the data? Should we now all take huge amounts of vitamin D to protect ourselves and our children from MS? Could high doses of vitamin D actually cure MS? First, a warning is in order. Very large quantities of vitamin D are not healthy. They can cause excessive amounts of calcium to accumulate in blood, and subsequently become deposited in lungs, kidney, heart, and blood vessels, causing considerable damage. Also, now going out into the blazing sun all the time, or frequently using sunbeds, is not a great idea either. The risk of developing skin cancer as a result of excessive exposure to ultraviolet light is well known. Instead, taking moderate amounts of extra vitamin D, especially in winter, is an excellent idea. Although it will not cure MS, it may well be of benefit to suppress its symptoms.

The daily recommended intake of vitamin D as a supplement is under debate. Typically, policy makers tend to recommend 200–400 International Units (IU) daily, which is the same as 5–10 micrograms. The UK Food Standards Agency, for example, does so. Yet, several experts in the field have recently called upon health authorities to re-examine the issue. Based on new research and insights, authorities are encouraged to update their recommendations for daily intake. Current research indicates that the generally recommended quantities will not have very much effect at all, raising blood levels of vitamin D only marginally, but not up to the 'safe' levels of about 100 nmol/L. To achieve real protective effects, daily extra intake of about 2000 IU of vitamin D makes more sense for most people. In combination with routine exposure to sunlight (exposing the face and arms for about 15 minutes per day) without using sunbeds or spending weeks on the beach, this should be enough to supply your body with what it needs. It is estimated that 2000 IU of supplementary vitamin D every day will generally raise blood levels up to around the required safe levels. Upper limits for vitamin D intake, levels at which it will start to lead to toxic effects of calcium, are estimated at around 10,000 IU per day. These levels must therefore certainly be avoided. Given that people differ in body weight, feeding patterns, and sunbathing habits, which all influence vitamin D levels in your body, it is therefore recommended to not go beyond taking 2000 IU (or 50 micrograms) of extra vitamin D per day. It should do. For people with MS, this may well reduce the chance of developing another relapse by about 50%. This effect is similar to that of most MS drugs. As stated before, the protective effect of vitamin D adds to that of MS drugs. Having regular MS medication should therefore be no reason for anyone with MS to ignore the benefits of vitamin D. And everyone should give it to their children too.

Further reading

Farinotti M, Simi S, Di Pietrantonj C, *et al.* (2007) Dietary interventions for multiple sclerosis. *Cochrane Database Syst Rev* 24: CD004192.

Kampman MT and Brustad M (2008) Vitamin D: a candidate for the environmental effect in multiple sclerosis—observations from Norway. *Neuroepidemiology* 30: 140–6.

Mora JR, Iwata M, and von Andrian UH (2008) Vitamin effects on the immune system: vitamins A and D take centre stage. *Nat Rev Immunol* 8: 685–98.

Namaka M, Crook A, Doupe A, *et al.* (2008) Examining the evidence: complementary adjunctive therapies for multiple sclerosis. *Neurol Res* 30: 710–19.

Ucelli A, Laroni A, and Freedman MS (2011) Mesenchymal stem cells for the treatment of multiple sclerosis and other neurological diseases. *Lancet Neurol* 10: 649–56.

Useful websites

Multiple Sclerosis Society

http://www.mssociety.org.uk

Multiple Sclerosis Society, Getting involved in clinical trials

http://www.mssociety.org.uk/ms-research/get-involved-research/get-involved-in-clinical-trials

National Multiple Sclerosis Society

http://www.nationalmssociety.org

National Multiple Sclerosis Society, Clinical trials

http://www.nationalmssociety.org/research/clinical-trials/index.aspx

MS Trust StayingSmart

http://www.stayingsmart.org.uk

Index